AF675103

Manual of

Vaginal Hysterectomy

Manual of
Vaginal Hysterectomy

Editors

SN Tripathy

KC Mahapatra

SK Giri

RM Saraogi

Narahari Agasthi

JAYPEE *The Health Sciences Publisher*

New Delhi | London | Panama

Jaypee Brothers Medical Publishers (P) Ltd

Headquarters

Jaypee Brothers Medical Publishers (P) Ltd
4838/24, Ansari Road, Daryaganj
New Delhi 110 002, India
Phone: +91-11-43574357
Fax: +91-11-43574314
Email: jaypee@jaypeebrothers.com

Overseas Offices

J.P. Medical Ltd
83 Victoria Street, London
SW1H 0HW (UK)
Phone: +44-20 317 08910
Fax: +44 (0)20 3008 6180
Email: info@jpmedpub.com

Jaypee-Highlights Medical Publishers Inc
City of Knowledge, Bld. 235, 2nd floor, Clayton
Panama City, Panama
Phone: +1 507-301-0496
Fax: +1 507-301-0499
Email: cservice@jphmedical.com

Jaypee Brothers Medical Publishers (P) Ltd
17/1-B Babar Road, Block-B, Shyamoli
Mohammadpur, Dhaka-1207
Bangladesh
Mobile: +08801912003485
Email: jaypeedhaka@gmail.com

Jaypee Brothers Medical Publishers (P) Ltd
Bhotahity, Kathmandu, Nepal
Phone: +977-9741283608
Email: Kathmandu@jaypeebrothers.com

Website: www.jaypeebrothers.com
Website: www.jaypeedigital.com

Inquiries for bulk sales may be solicited at: jaypee@jaypeebrothers.com

Manual of Vaginal Hysterectomy

First Edition: **2018**

ISBN 978-93-5270-368-5

Printed at: Samrat Offset Pvt. Ltd.

Contributors

Haresh U Doshi

Kurush P Paghdiwalla

Meenakshi Patel

Mohan A Gadam

Nirmal N Gujarathi

Preeti D Galvankar

Rajkumar H Shah

Ramesh Desale

Raut VS

Sahu RR

RM Saraogi

Shirish S Sheth

Vidya Pancholia

Message

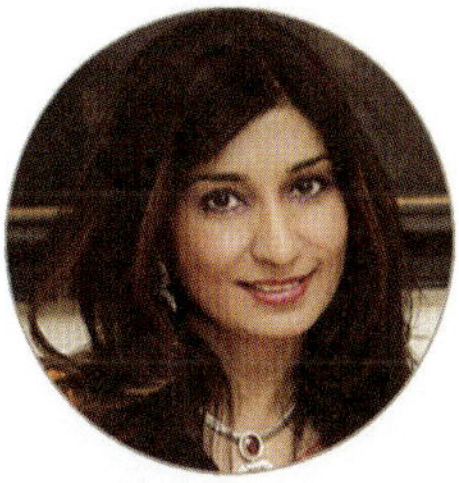

Rishma Dhillon Pai
MD DNB FCPS DGO FICOG
President, FOGSI—2017
Consultant Gynecologist
Jaslok Hospital, Lilavati Hospital and Hinduja Healthcare (Khar),
Bloom IVF Centre,
The Every Woman Clinic,
Mumbai, Maharashtra, India

"Wisdom.... comes not from age, but from education and learning."
Anton Chekhov

Life is a continuous process of learning. Especially in the field of medicine, which is constantly changing, it is very important to keep oneself abreast with the latest developments. It is heartening to note that academic workshop manuals are being released at the AICOG, Bhubaneswar, Odisha, India, for the benefit of the participating delegates and present varied updates in the field. Many different Manuals are being released on important subjects such as *3D Laparoscopy and Operative Oncology, Genetics, Fetal Medicine and Color Doppler, Postpartum Hemorrhage and High-Risk Pregnancy, Hysteroscopy,* etc.

I thank all the authors, for their immense contributions in building up the content for the manuals for Federation of Obstetric and Gynaecological Societies of India (FOGSI) by sharing their rich experiences in the field. These will be a big help to young gynecologists, who are still acquiring skills in various aspects of obstetrics and gynecology and a quick update for the seniors.

I extend congratulations to the organizing team of the AICOG 2018 and the editors of these manuals and wish you all success for this mega event.

"You cannot open a book without learning something."
—Confucius

Message

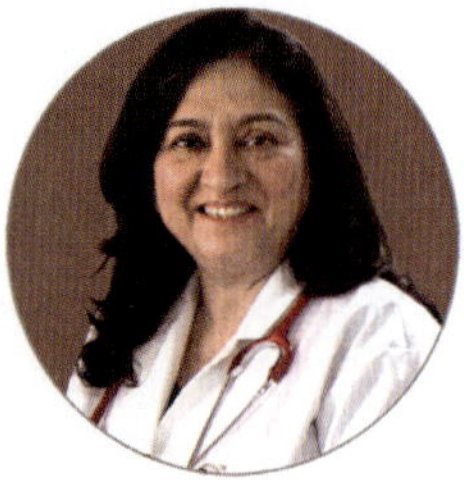

Jaideep Malhotra
MD FICMCH FICS FMAS FRCOG FICOG FRCPI FIAJAGO
Consultant ART (IVF)
President Elect, FOGSI—2018
Director, Rainbow IVF
Agra, Uttar Pradesh, India

"Education is greatest gift of life, it should never stop."

The subject of obstetrics and gynecology needs extreme proficiency as it deals with the medical specialties that focus on two different aspects. First one includes the care of pregnant women, the unborn baby, labor and delivery, as well as the immediate period following childbirth. Second aspect includes dealing with any ailment concerning the female reproductive organs. Hence, the manuals will help all those who are looking forward to gain excellence in the field of woman health. The manuals have tried to address all the issues a doctor needs.

With increasing expertise in all fields, the surgeon therefore while exercising a choice needs to follow the Hippocratic dictum—"*First, do no harm.*"

We are thankful to all those who have incorporated their contribution by providing chapters from their research and collected scientific material and have shared their fruitful experiences for the delegates of the workshop.

As a part of my agenda for 2018, I as FOGSI President 2018, plan to work actively on QED (Quality, Ethics and Dignity) among our profession and also work towards HER (Health, Empowerment and Respect) towards our patients.

"Knowledge is of no value unless you put it into practices."

Message

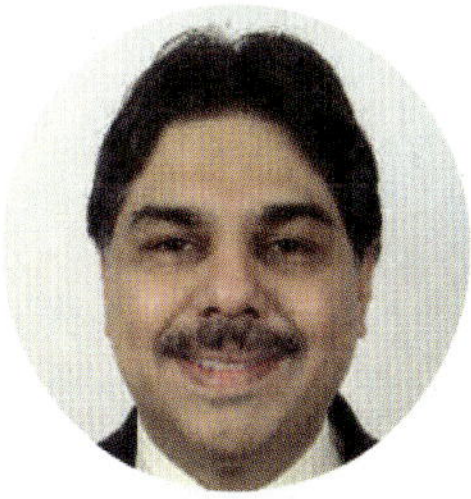

Hrishikesh Pai
Secretary General, FOGSI

It is my proud privilege to invite and welcome all delegates to the 61st All India Congress of Obstetrics and Gynaecology (AICOG) from 17th–21st January, 2018 at the Temple City of India, Bhubaneswar, Odisha, India.

It is propitious to note that the academic workshop manuals are being released which will reap beneficial reward to all the participating delegates.

I thank all the authors, for their immense contributions in building up the content for the manuals for Federation of Obstetric and Gynaecological Societies of India (FOGSI) by sharing their rich experiences in the field. These will be a big help to young gynecologists, who are still acquiring skills in various aspects of obstetrics and gynecology and a quick update for the seniors.

I forward my heartiest congratulations to all the contributors, the editors and the delegates of the workshop.

Message

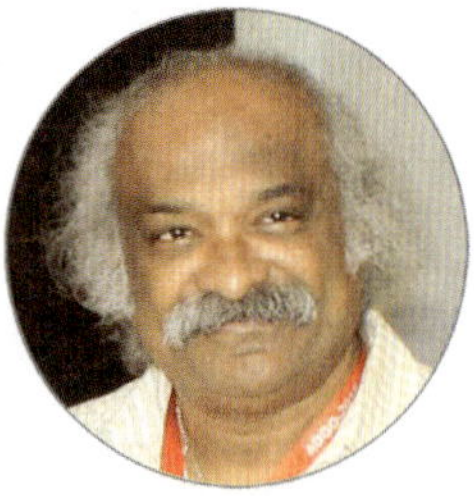

PC Mahapatra
Professor
Department of Obstetrics and Gynecology
SCB Medical College
Cuttack, Odisha, India
President, FOGSI—2011
Organising Chairperson

It is my proud privilege to invite and welcome all delegates to the 61st All India Congress of Obstetrics and Gynaecology (AICOG) from 17th–21st January, 2018 at the Temple City of India, Bhubaneswar, Odisha, India.

The five days of academic extravaganza will certainly enrich the scientific knowledge of all participating delegates and faculty. The precongress workshop on various aspects of this specialty will be held on 17th January 2018.

A quote by Edwin Louis Cole says that "*Winners are not those who never fail but those who never quit*" is apt for all the clinicians who are determined enough to see and overcome all the difficulties that are faced in the field of obstetrics and gynecology.

Today, with the advancement in the field of obstetrics and gynecology, everyone requires an in-depth knowledge of the complex subjects associated with the field so as to gain excellence in it.

This manual will prove to be a boon to all those who are associated with the field and wants to gain more knowledge in the subject matter.

Message

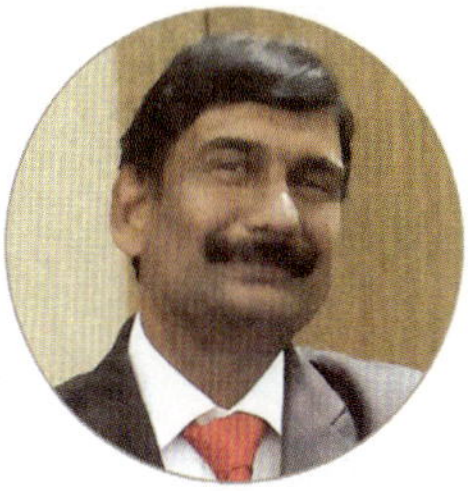

HP Pattanaik
Head
Department of Obstetrics and Gynecology
City Hospital
Cuttack, Odisha, India
Vice President, FOGSI—2009
Organising Secretary

Greetings from 61st AICOG 2018!

It is a matter of great pleasure to invite you all to 61st AICOG, from 17th–21st January, 2018 at the Temple City of India, Bhubaneswar, Odisha, India. The 11th Precongress workshops will be held on 17th January, 2018 in three medical colleges of Bhubaneswar.

It is propitious to note that the academic workshop manuals are being released which will reap beneficial reward to all the participating delegates.

It will also prove to be beneficial to the members of Federation of Obstetric and Gynaecological Societies of India (FOGSI), those who were unable to register themselves for the academic workshops.

I forward my heartiest congratulations to all the contributors, the editors and the delegates of the workshop.

Preface

Rapid progress in technology in all specialties of scientific world makes it necessary for individuals to attend meetings and workshops to stay abreast with advances. We in India are now fortunate to have opportunities as regular workshops, conferences are conducted in the length and breadth of the country. The most operation in Gynecology is hysterectomy. With the advent of laparoscopy and safer anesthesia protocols, abdominal route for hysterectomy is gradually decreasing. But this should not be a reason for decline in the vaginal approach for surgery.

The female pelvis can be accessed easily either through the natural orifice, i.e. vagina or through other surgically created incision. The vaginal approach has been the hallmark of the gynecological surgeon. Every gynecologist should include vaginal surgeries and especially vaginal hysterectomy in their armamentarium to serve their patients better as the patient is, and should be the only concern, for a surgeon, for carrying out a hysterectomy, by the route that is most optimal for her. Hence, it is imperative that one has operative expertise to use for the best outcomes, morbidity and patient's recovery.

The advantages of hysterectomy vaginally usually outweigh advantages of alternative methods of hysterectomy. Abdominal hysterectomy in particular invites incisional hernia, more so, in Indian women with poor abdominal wall strength. Oldest method of access, i.e. vaginal is best method of access to remove uterus whenever possible. The American College of Obstetrics and gynaecology and Cochrane database review suggests that vaginal hysterectomy is safest and preferable route when compared to abdominal and laparoscopic route. It is most cost effective in terms of operative time, hospital stay and overall postoperative morbidity.

At any stage of the surgery by the vaginal route (VH), if the situation warrants a change to a laparoscopic and/or abdominal route, there should be no hesitation to do so or have a false sense of ego, which will affect the patient adversely. An action taken as 'TRIAL VH' in the patient's best interest's invites admiration and sometimes failure to complete the procedure as planned vaginally. It is comparable to a trial forceps delivery in obstetrics. 'TRIAL' will considerably reduce the number of abdominal hysterectomies or abdominal access, enhance the operator's experience and judgment. When in doubt or anxious, laparoscopic evaluation will help. It is 'diagnostic' evaluation of intraperitoneal adhesions and assesses fitness for the vaginal route. It is vastly different from laparoscopically assisted vaginal hysterectomy (LAVH). Other surgeries performed by vaginal route are VVF repair, vault prolapse repair, colpocleisis etc. We have stalwarts in the workshop to elaborate and discuss about the operative procedure.

Reading makes you ready, seeing makes you steady, practice makes you perfect.

Wokshops does all this and much more. We are really happy to bring out a manual of this workshop.

"Let sugery fit to the patient rather than patient fit to surgery."

Editors

Contents

Chapter 1

Surgical Anatomy of the Pelvis: As Applicable for Vaginal Hysterectomy

Rajkumar H Shah

INTRODUCTION

The uterus is a unique organ as it lies suspended in the pelvic cavity, by its elastic supports. These supports allow the uterus to get distended during pregnancy and involute back to its original location. These supports require to be cut and transfixed whenever a surgery for its removal is done. These supports are enumerated below:

- *Upper tier supports*:
  - The round ligaments
  - Broad ligament with intervening pelvic cellular tissues
  - Endopelvic fascia covering the uterus
- *Middle tier supports*:
  - Cervicovaginal junction—important direct support (fibromuscular tissue surrounding the vessels and nerves)
  - Pelvic cellular tissues (connective tissue and smooth muscles) through which blood vessels and nerve supply pass through from lateral pelvic wall, condense surrounding them and give direct support
  - The condensation of the tissues surrounding the supravaginal cervix and vagina down to the superior layer of the fascia covering the cervicovaginal junction
  - The condensation and reinforcement by plain muscles to form ligaments—Mackenrodt's, uterosacral and pubocervical.
- *Inferior tier*: Musculofascial tone of the hollow vagina by the fascial condensation at the vault and by the pelvic floor.

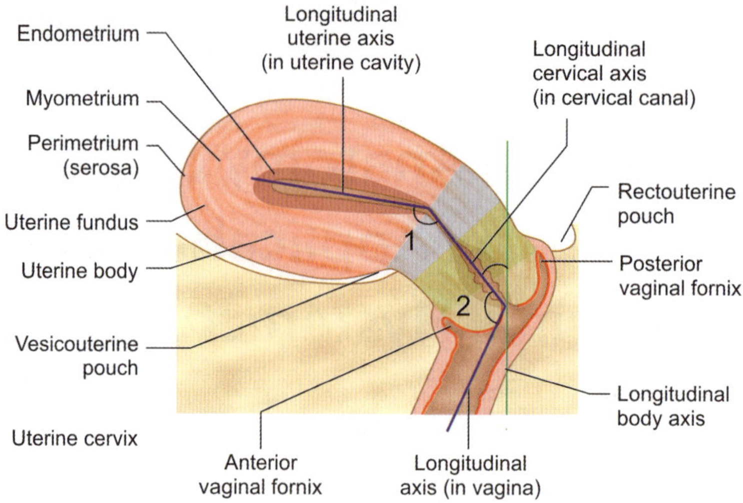

Fig. 1: Uterus: a unique organ and its representation.

The uterus and its supports are covered by the visceral peritoneum which gets reflected anteriorly from the roof of the bladder onto the anterior abdominal wall forming the parietal peritoneum and posteriorly onto the rectum reaching lower into the pelvis forming the cul-de-sac (pouch of Douglas). At hysterectomy, once these pouches are rendered open, the blood supply to the uterus can be approached, on the lateral aspects (Fig. 1).

BLOOD SUPPLY OF THE UTERUS (FIGS. 2 AND 3)

Whenever a surgical extirpation of an organ is planned, it is imperative to know the intricacies of its blood supply. The uterus is no exception. In fact, when a vaginal hysterectomy is done for a bulky uterus, there are ways and means of morcellation of the uterus and at this point in time, knowing the blood supply of the uterus is very important.

The blood supply is mainly from:

- The uterine artery, arising as a branch of the internal iliac artery and then dividing into the ascending and descending branch, and
- The ovarian artery arising from the aorta, and anastomosing with the ascending uterine, within the broad ligament.

The ascending uterine artery gives off arcuate vessels at regular intervals from the lateral walls to the midline and joins up with other vessels from the opposite side. This makes the midline least vascular.

In view of the blood supply arising from both the sides, it is essential to go symmetrically to impede the blood vessels by use of clamps or sutures and prevent blood loss.

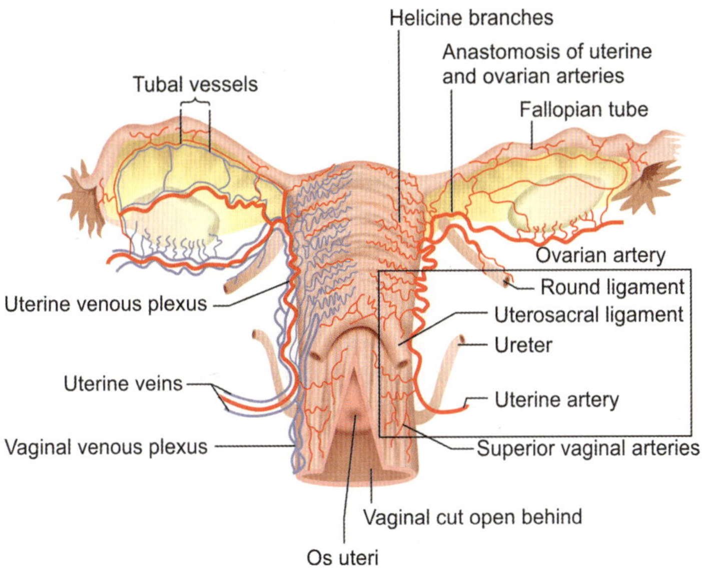

Fig. 2: Vaginal hysterectomy.

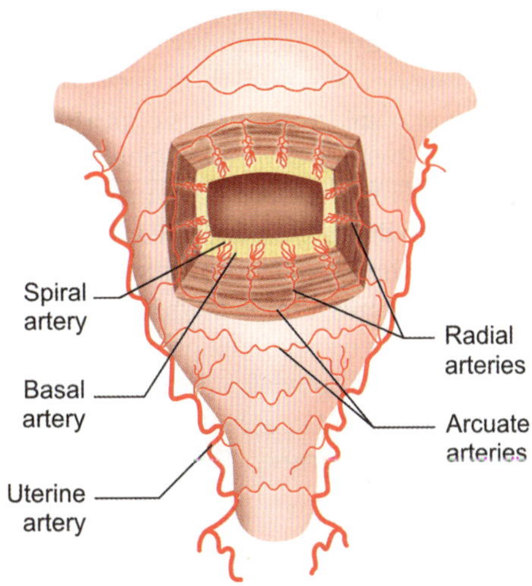

Fig. 3: Blood supply of the arteries.

It is essential to deliver the fundus of the uterus from the anterior pouch, to maintain the anatomical relations. If delivered from the posterior pouch, the normal anatomy could get distorted, but can still be done at times, if deemed necessary.

APPLIED SURGICAL ANATOMY

The incision on the cervix anteriorly has to be planned to avoid injury to the urinary bladder. Especially, in prolapse uterus, too low an incision would result in unnecessary extensive dissection before reaching the anterior pouch. A very high incision may be easier to approach the anterior pouch but may lead to sacrificing a large portion of the vagina, compromising the effective length of the vagina leading to sexual problems postsurgery.

The anterior pouch can be rendered open in three simple steps. First, placing the anterior incision on the cervix. Second, sharp dissection and picking up the vesicouterine ligament. This can be incised, exposing the anterior pouch. Third, picking up the peritoneum between two hemostats and incising the peritoneum to render the anterior pouch open.

The posterior incision is taken in different ways. An Ellis forceps could be placed on the posterior vaginal wall, grasping the underlying peritoneum of the pouch and opening it in one swift incision with a scissor. The only disadvantage of this method is that it compromises a large portion of the vagina, reducing its effective length. A second method would be to do it identical to the anterior pouch, by incising the vagina and dissecting till the posterior peritoneum is reached and then incising it between two Ellis forceps. This maintains a decent length of the vagina, but could cause bleeding due to excessive dissection, once the effect of injected adrenaline solution wears off.

Once, both the pouches are opened, it is essential to apply clamps or place sutures in such a manner that both the leaves of the broad ligament are included, so as to take care of all the branches of the uterine artery.

When a bulky uterus is being delivered vaginally, there are various ways the uterus is morcellated—bisection or decompressing by Lash's technique. These involve clamping and ligating the uterine arteries and then proceeding with the morcellation procedure. Once the uterine arteries are obliterated, the morcellation procedure becomes almost bloodless.

Lastly, if the adnexa is to be excised, the proximal part of the infundibulo-pelvic ligament is identified and special clamps applied before excision.

It is essential to maintain a good length of the vagina at surgery, for allowing satisfactory coital function, postsurgery. This can be done by adhering to the suggestions made above as also, suspending the vault of the vagina to the adnexal stumps.

Chapter 2

Preoperative Preparations, Postoperative Care and Indications

Preeti D Galvankar, Nirmal N Gujarathi

INTRODUCTION

More than 30 million surgeries are performed every year, world over and out of those one million patients suffer a postoperative complication. A gynecologist assumes responsibility for assessing a patient's clinical status to identify modifiable risk factors and prevent perioperative morbidity. We should also be prepared to diagnose and manage such complications.[1]

Oldest method of access, i.e. vaginal is best method of access to remove uterus whenever possible. The American College of Obstetrics and Gynecology (ACOG) and Cochrane database review suggests that vaginal hysterectomy is safest and preferable route when compared to abdominal and laparoscopic route. It is most cost-effective in terms of operative time, hospital stay and overall postoperative morbidity.[2]

PREOPERATIVE PATIENT EVALUATION

Preoperative preparation is important for two purposes:

1. It detects comorbidities that require further evaluation and optimization to prevent further complications
2. It allows improved use of resources.

Pulmonary System

Risk factors:

- *Procedure related*: Intraoperative stimulation of viscera, muscle disruption and pain may limit respiratory efforts, which leads to atelectasis. General anesthesia longer than 3 hours can increase risk of postoperative pulmonary complications.

- *Patient related*: Age more than 60, smoking more than 20 pack year, chronic obstructive pulmonary disease (COPD), obstructive sleep apnea, obesity [body mass index (BMI) >30], asthma.
- *Postoperative comorbidities*: Atelectasis, pneumonia and exacerbation of chronic lung disease.

Prevention: Pulmonary function test prior to surgery, lung expansion modalities like deep breathing exercises, incentive spirometry and early ambulation.

Cardiac System

Risk factors: Valvular heart disease, heart failure, arrhythmias, and hypertension.

Preventive strategies: Perioperative beta-blockers, coronary revascularization, and anemia correction.

Hepatic System

Liver plays important role in drug metabolism, protein synthesis, coagulation factors and excretion of endogenous compounds.

Risk factors: History of jaundice in recent past, recent travel history, alcohol consumption and exposure to hepatotoxic medications, acute and chronic hepatitis, anemia.

In such patients, in addition to liver function tests, coagulation profiles to be done.

Preventive strategy: Gastroenterological evaluation and specialist opinion prior to surgery should be mandatory.

Renal System

Kidneys are involved in excretion of metabolic waste, hematologic processes and fluid and electrolyte balance.

Risk factors: Chronic kidney disease, anemia due to kidney disorders, electrolyte imbalance.

Preventive strategy: Electrolyte correction, dialysis prior to surgery in required cases, anemia correction, nephrologist involvement.

Hematologic Evaluation

Risk factors: Anemia, coagulopathies and patients on anticoagulants, autologous blood donation: Preoperative autologous donation and salvage autologous transfusions.

Preventive strategy: Anemia correction prior to surgery by iron, multivitamin supplementations, in emergency cases by blood transfusion, correction of coagulopathies.

Patients on anticoagulants, needs to maintain international normalized ration (INR) around 1.5 prior to surgery. Anticoagulant bridging protocols to be used while shifting patient from oral to intravenous (IV)/subcutaneous (SC) heparin and postsurgery. The INR to be monitored and maintained between two and three postsurgery.[3]

Endocrine Evaluation

Risk factors: Diabetes mellitus, and thyroid disorders.

Increased postoperative morbidity has been associated with poor preoperative glycemic control (blood glucose levels >200 mg/dL and HbA1c >7).[4]

Hyperthyroidism can lead to thyroid storm perioperatively. Patients with goiter can lead to airway compromise.

Preventive strategy: Vigilant preoperative risk assessment for women affected with diabetes mellitus of long-standing is essential, as we are likely to encounter vascular, neurologic, cardiac and renal dysfunction. Preoperatively euglycemic status to be achieved in all such patients.

Management goal for hyperthyroid and hypothyroid patients is to achieve euthyroid status prior to surgery.

SURGICAL CONSIDERATIONS

Infection prophylaxis: As per ACOG 2014a, recommendations, single dose of antibiotic at anesthesia induction to be given. Additional doses should be considered for obese individuals, longer duration of surgery, blood loss more than 1,500 mL. In our setup, we are using cefazolin 1 g single dose prior to surgery and in urogynecological procedures gentamicin or quinolone and metronidazole to be added.

POSTOPERATIVE CARE

Most of the postsurgical problems can be avoided by proper preoperative risk assessment and preventive strategies. However, in spite of due care complications may still develop which need to be treated in time.

Pain Management

Poor postoperative pain control can lead to prolonged hospital stay, patient dissatisfaction and increased cost of procedure.

Major classes of nonopioid analgesics are paracetamol and nonsteroidal anti-inflammatory drugs (NSAIDs). Advantages of giving postoperative analgesics are: reduced opiates requirements, decrease incidence of postoperative nausea and vomiting (PONV), postoperative pain. Nonopioids are generally well tolerated with low risk of serious side effects.

Opiates are primary choice for managing moderate to severe pain, despite of common side effects like respiratory depression, nausea and vomiting.

Fluid and Electrolytes

Daily fluid requirement of average adult is 30 mL/kg/day. Thus, postoperatively crystalloid fluids are used for maintenance, as they increase interstitial volume and do not affect plasma volume. Most commonly used crystalloids are lactated Ringer's solution and isotonic saline. Postoperatively potassium levels should be maintained to avoid paralytic ileus.

Postoperative Nausea and Vomiting

Postoperative nausea and vomiting is most common complain which can be controlled with use of antiemetics like benzamides (metoclopramide), phenothiazines group (prochlorperazine, promethazine) and serotonin antagonists (ondansetron).

Deep Vein Thrombosis Prophylaxis

Deep vein thrombosis (DVT) prophylaxis should be offered to high-risk patients like obese, past history of DVT, on anticoagulants and bedridden patients (delayed ambulation). Different forms of DVT prophylaxis are: use of heparin, intermittent pneumatic compression devices, thromboembolic device (TED) stockings, oral anticoagulants and physiotherapy.

Bowel Function and Diet

Nowadays early resumption of diet has shown to improve gut motility, decrease stasis/ileus, increase splanchnic blood flow, stimulate gastrointestinal (GI) hormone secretions which shortens postoperative ileus.

Bladder Care

Indwelling self-retaining catheter for first 24 hours is important from monitoring of intake and output balance. Patency of catheter should be monitored especially in cases of anterior colporrhaphy.

INDICATIONS AND CONTRAINDICATIONS FOR VAGINAL HYSTERECTOMY

Indications

- Uterovaginal prolapse
- Abnormal uterine bleeding
- Fibroids up to 12 weeks size
- Adenomyosis
- Fibroid polyps
- Premalignant conditions of cervix and endometrium.

Contraindications

Relative Contraindications

- Uterus size greater than 12 weeks
- Benign adnexal pathology
- Broad ligament fibroid.

Absolute Contraindications

- Uterus size greater than 20 weeks
- Inaccessible cervix
- Cervical and endometrial malignancy
- Adnexal malignancy
- Previous successfully repaired vesicovaginal fistula and rectovaginal fistula.

REFERENCES

1. Mangano DT. Perioperative medicine: NHLBI working group deliberations and recommendations. J Cardiothorac Vasc Anesth. 2004;18:1-6.
2. Nieboer TE, Johnson N, Lethaby A, et al. Surgical approach to hysterectomy for benign gynaecological disease. Cochrane database Syst Rev. 2009;(3):CD003677.
3. Douketis JD, Spyropoulos AC, Spencer FA, et al. Perioperative management of antithrombotic therapy: Antithrombotic Therapy and Prevention of Thrombosis, 9th ed: Americal College of Chest Physicians Evidence-Based Clinical Practice Guidelines. Chest. 2012;141(2 Suppl):e326S-50S.
4. Dronge AS, Perkal MF, Kancir S, et al. Long-term glycemic control and postoperative infectious complications. Arch Surg. 2006;141:375-80.

Chapter 3

Vaginal Surgeries in Case of Previous Abdominal Surgeries

Shirish S Sheth, Kurush P Paghdiwalla

"Some of the iatrogenic contraindications are truly indications to progress for others. As experience increases some of the contraindications regress".

Sheth Shirish S

INTRODUCTION

Vaginal surgery, commonly hysterectomy after previous abdomino-pelvic surgery can test the surgical skills of the operating surgeon to the limit.[1]

The patient is, and should be the only concern, for a surgeon, for carrying out a hysterectomy, by the route that is most optimal for her. Hence, it is imperative that one has operative expertise to use for the best outcomes, morbidity and patient's recovery.

When in doubt or anxious, laparoscopic evaluation will help. It is 'diagnostic' evaluation of intraperitoneal adhesions and assesses fitness for the vaginal route. It is vastly different from laparoscopically assisted vaginal hysterectomy (LAVH).

At any stage of the surgery by the vaginal route (VH), if the situation warrants a change to a laparoscopic and/or abdominal route, there should be no hesitation to do so or have a false sense of ego, and affect the patient adversely. An action taken as 'TRIAL VH' in the patient's best interest's invites admiration and sometimes failure to complete the procedure as planned vaginally. It is comparable to a trial forceps delivery in obstetrics. 'TRIAL' will considerably reduce the number of abdominal hysterectomies or abdominal access, enhance the operator's experience and judgment.

The advantages of hysterectomy vaginally usually outweigh advantages of alternative methods of hysterectomy. Abdominal hysterectomy in particular invites incisional hernia, more so, in Indian women with poor abdominal wall strength.

CESAREAN SECTION(S) IN PAST

Women, who have undergone any of one or more cesarean section(s), myomectomy, suspension procedures and genital tuberculosis, may have anterior adhesions.[2] One of the techniques that the author prefers for more than two decades and finds very useful in circumventing these adhesions is to use the anatomically available lateral window, surgical window or the uterocervical broad ligament space; this allows access to the vesicouterine fold of the peritoneum.[3,4] Familiarity with this surgical window will reduce laparoscopic as well as abdominal hysterectomies as bladder trauma (in accessing vesicouterine peritoneum) is the main deterrent or inhibitor.

Laparoscopic or abdominal hysterectomy is indicated when vaginal hysterectomy is contraindicated. When the clinical findings are not conducive, especially in the early years of practice, gynecologists may reassess them by examination under anesthesia and if doubt persists, take full advantage of laparoscopic assistance in the form of evaluation and/or operation to complete the hysterectomy vaginally. A Pfannenstiel scar on the abdomen for C-section(s) in past indicates a high level of surgical principles, and a cleaner peritoneal cavity.

Currently large number, at times even 50% of deliveries are carried out by cesarean section in many countries. With this trend likely to continue and flourish, Gynecologists will have to increasingly face the problem at hysterectomy in almost alternate patient with one or multiple cesarean sections in the past. In women with C-sections in past, gynecologist and sonologist must also look for clinical cervico fundal and sonographic signs respectively.[5,6] Previous vaginal delivery before and more so, after a caesarean section would make the vaginal route easier. A patient who has undergone a cesarean section in past without vaginal delivery before or after is vaginally nullipara, though multiparous abdominally.[7]

SURGICAL TECHNIQUE

The surgeon requires access to both pouches and familiarity with the 'landmarks'. It is not obligatory to open the peritoneum at the start of surgery, as long as the bladder and rectum are well separated, protected and kept out of harm's way by the bladder retractor and speculum respectively. Well seen peritoneum may even be opened after the uterine vessels are well secured. It is also worth learning the clamp-less technique[8,9] for VH as it is particularly useful when space is at a premium. The use of a specially designed, fibreoptic, illuminated speculum and/or bladder retractors can felicitate.

The most common surgical procedures performed on the uterus are: cesarean section, myomectomy and hysterotomy, demanding extra care, but do not constitute a contraindication (Table 1).[9] Ventrofixation, an obsolete procedure, contraindicates vaginal hysterectomy as a result of a mechanical factor except in very experienced hands.

- Sling operations for prolapse including Shirodkar's, also make vaginal hysterectomy difficult. An experienced vaginal surgeon will be able to cope without laparoscopic assistance
- Operations performed on the tubes, ovaries, and broad ligament tissues can give rise to a few flimsy adhesions close to the upper pedicle, which are easily separable and do not hinder surgery. History of tubal sterilization or even ectopic pregnancy is not a contraindication and should not deter the surgeon
- Operations performed on structures or organs other than the genital tract, such as those involving the intestines, gallbladder, and urinary tract (but not the bladder), are not contraindications to vaginal hysterectomy. Just as history of vaginal hysterectomy does not contraindicate cholecystectomy, in no way history of cholecystectomy and allied should ever contraindicate hysterectomy via vaginal route. Surgery on bladder and/or rectum in past demand extra careful evaluation of surgical site, clinical findings and surgeon's access.

Table 1: The categories of previous surgeries and possibility of VH[9]

Type of surgery	*Possibility of vaginal hysterectomy*
Operations performed on uterus: Cesarean section(s), hysterotomy, myomectomy Ventrosuspension	Possible with extra care. To go by clinical findings plus EUA
Abdominal sling operations for prolapse (Shirodkar's, Purandare's, and Virkud's sling)	Possible with advanced level of skills
Operation on structures or organs other than the genital tract, e.g. adhesiolysis/ small intestines/gallbladder	Possible with ease
Previous rectosigmoid resection with low rectal anastomosis	Possible with extra care
Operations performed on tubes, ovaries, broad ligaments	Possible
Operations on urinary tract: Bladder, e.g. successful VVF repair done in region of cervix or proximal vagina. Previous midurethral slings	Contraindicated Possible with ease

(EUA: examination under anesthesia; VVF: vesiocovaginal fistula)

Previous surgery in the vaginal region is not itself a contraindication to vaginal hysterectomy but deserves extra care and dexterity.

Cervical amputation and Fothergill's operation, previous vesicovaginal fistula (VVF), and rectovaginal fistula (RVF) repairs all distort the anatomy considerably in the genital area. To use the vaginal route in these cases would be tantamount to inviting bladder and/or bowel injury, except in the hands of an exceptionally few, truly advanced vaginal surgeons. The use of laparoscopic assistance from well experienced laparoscopists or the abdominal route is preferred.

Previous abdominopelvic surgery is enough to put off the gynecologists particularly, the one who is less inclined towards the vaginal route though per se it does not contraindicate the vaginal route. It is an easy excuse to avoid vaginal route. However, the type of the previous operations is the deciding factor.

Some of these cases can be guided by examination under anesthesia (EUA) to decide on the use of laparoscopy to free adhesions and/or confirm the absence of peritoneal adhesions. The presence of any adhesion that makes the uterus inseparable or that risks traumatizing a hollow organ should be an indication to abandon the vaginal route and complete the operation with help of laparoscope or abdominally.

REFERENCES

1. Nichols DH, Randall CL. Vaginal Surgery, 3rd eduction. Baltimore, MA: Williams & Wilkins, 1983; pp188-9.
2. Sheth SS, Malpani AN. Vaginal hysterectomy following previous caesarean section. Int J Gynecol Obstet. 1995;50(2):165-9.
3. Sizzi O, Paparella P, Bonito C, et al. Laparoscopic assistance after vaginal hysterectomy and unsuccessful access to the ovaries or failed uterine mobilization: changing trends. JSLS. 2004;8:339-46.
4. Paparella P, Sizzi O, Rossetti A, et al. Vaginal hysterectomy in generally considered contraindications to vaginal surgery. Arch Gynecol Obstet. 2004; 270(2):104-9.
5. Sheth SS, Goyal MV, Shah N. Uterocervical displacement following adhesions after caesarean section. J Gynecol Surg. 1997;13:143-7.
6. Sheth SS, Shah NM, Varaiya D. A sonographic and clinical sign to detect specific adhesions following caesarean section. J Gynecol Surgery. 2008; 24: 27-35.
7. Sheth SS, Paghdiwalla KP. Hysterectomy: choice of surgical approach. FOGSI Text Book Obst-Gynec. 2013.
8. Sheth SS. Vaginal hysterectomy. In: Studd J (Ed). Progress in obstetrics and gynecology, 10th eduction. London: Churchill Livingstone; 1993, pp. 317-40.
9. Sheth SS. Vaginal or abdominal hysterectomy? In: Sheth SS (Ed). Vaginal hysterectomy, Second Edition. New Delhi, India: Jaypee Brothers Medical Publishers (P) Ltd; 2014; 273-93.

Chapter 4

Vaginal Surgeries with Adnexal Pathology

Raut VS, Sahu RR

INTRODUCTION

The most gynecological surgeries are hysterectomy, ovarian cystectomy, myomectomy, and pelvic endometriosis. With the advent of laparoscopy and safer anesthesia protocols, abdominal route for gynecological pathology has been gradually decreasing. But this should not be a reason for decline in the vaginal approach for surgery especially hysterectomy.

The female pelvis can be accessed easily either through the natural orifice, i.e. vagina or through other surgically created incision. The vaginal approach has been the hallmark of the gynecological surgeon. Every gynecologist should include vaginal surgeries and especially vaginal hysterectomy in their armamentarium to serve their patients better.

"Man learns as he lives and experience is the greatest teacher in the world" (Swami Vivekananda).

When uterine pathology is associated with any adnexal pathology like ovarian cyst, hydrosalpinx, paraovarian cyst, broad ligament fibroid, the gynecologist review their decision of vaginal approach for surgery.

Maresh MJ, et al. 2002 showed that, in women aged 55–60 years, oophorectomy was carried out in 92% during abdominal hysterectomy, 96.6% during laparoscopically assisted vaginal hysterectomy (LAVH), and only 9.4% during vaginal hysterectomy. This indicates that most of the gynecologists are not comfortable to remove the adnexal mass vaginally.[1]

Vaginal adnexal surgery can be considered in cases like:

- Mobile benign ovarian teratoma
- Simple serous ovarian cyst
- Non-adherent endometriotic cyst

- Cervical intraepithelial neoplasia (CIN) and stage IA1—stromal invasion less than 3 mm and no evidence of lymphovascular involvement
- Carcinoma of endometrium International Federation of Gynecology and Obstetrics (FIGO) Stage 1A—no or less than half myometrial invasion.

The exclusion criteria for vaginal surgery for hysterectomy or adnexal mass removal or vaginal colpotomy are as follows:

- Suspicion of malignancy; frozen section not available
- Adherent adnexal mass
- Obliterated cul-de-sac
- History of grade 3/4 endometriosis
- History of surgical repair of rectovaginal fistula or vescicovaginal fistula
- Active pelvic inflammatory disease
- Presence of vaginal infection
- Unmarried or sexually inactive women and narrow vagina
- Lack of operator's experience in vaginal surgery.

As experience of the surgeon in vaginal surgery increases, many contraindications become relative.

TECHNIQUE FOR VAGINAL SURGERY FOR ADNEXAL MASSES

The presence of uterine descent, as well as mobility of the uterus makes the fallopian tubes and ovaries more accessible vaginally.

If the infundibulopelvic ligament is accessible, the clamp is applied close to the adnexa, the ureter being 3 cm^3 or more away from the clamp. The infundibulopelvic ligament can be made prominent by applying gentle traction over the ovary with the help of Babcock's forceps and brought more medially. Gentle traction will prevent ligament tear, bleeding, and also help to place the suture beyond the clamp.

If only oophorectomy is planned, then the clamp is applied only on the meso-ovarium. The access to the meso-ovarium is easier than the infundibulopelvic ligament.

If salpingo-oophorectomy has been planned along with vaginal hysterectomy, then clamping and ligating the round ligament separately, 3–5 cm away from the uterus, will help to reach the infundibulopelvic ligament easily.

In some cases, especially in nondescent vaginal hysterectomy with bilateral salpingo-oophorectomy, keeping the cornual attachment intact makes it easier to access the infundibulopelvic ligament. The uterus helps to apply traction over the meso-ovarium and infundibulopelvic ligament. On the other hand, in larger uteri-like more than 12 weeks size, it is advisable to clamp the cornual structures first, remove the uterus and then approach the infundibulopelvic ligaments.

A specially designed clamp by Dr Shirish Sheth, which has a terminal 1 inch curve, helps in ensuring that the pedicle is securely grasped, and also provides better visualization while placing the ligature.[2,3] Instead of a Kocher clamp for infundibulopelvic ligament, a long curved artery forceps or a Mixter forceps can also be used.

Better vaginal exposure can be provided by placing the patient in steep Trendelenburg position and roller gauze pack to keep the omentum and intestines away.

In certain cases, using Deaver retractor, adequate light-like fiberoptic light source and an experienced assistant are of help to the surgeon to operate better.

Dr Shirish Sheth has published his work over two decades, where he has operated 750 vaginal hysterectomies with oophorectomies with no ureteral or bowel injuries and no postoperative hemorrhage.[2]

Dr Shirish Sheth has operated 166 women for vaginal hysterectomy with benign adnexal masses. In eight patients, laparotomy was needed due to malignancy reported on frozen section (three patients) and tubo-ovarian dense adhesions (five patients).[4,5]

The size of an ovarian cyst is not by itself a limiting factor, as the cyst can usually be aspirated and then excised. If the ovarian cyst is large and unilocular, it can be aspirated with a needle attached to the suction machine, to avoid spillage. The ovarian cyst wall can be delivered out with Babcock's forceps or a stay suture over the meso-ovarian ligament may also be helpful for traction.

TRANSVAGINAL EXTRACTION THROUGH POSTERIOR COLPOTOMY

During the past two decades, laparoscopy has become the most common route of gynecological surgeries especially hysterectomy and ovarian cystectomy.

The well-known advantages of laparoscopic procedures are smaller abdominal scars, better exposure of pelvic anatomy and lesser postoperative pain and intra-abdominal adhesions and shorter postoperative hospital stay. But, one of the most important disadvantages or downside of endoscopic surgery is the retrieval of surgical specimens like large myomas, dermoid ovarian cyst, and solid ovarian tumors intact from the small ports. Transvaginal extraction through posterior colpotomy should ensure the removal of surgical specimen intact (if possible) or with concomitant preservation of its integrity to avoid intra-abdominal spillage of potentially infected or malignant tissues.

After the specimen is separated from its abdominal and pelvis attachments, it is placed in an endobag. The pouch of Douglas can be opened transversely under laparoscopic guidance or vaginally and the closed end of the endobag is delivered through the vagina. The opening in endobag should cover the complete vulva, so as to prevent spillage and contamination with possibly infected specimen or malignant cells. If morcellation is required, it can be done within the endobag.

Stefano Uccella, et al. 2013 from Department of Gynecology, Italy, published a retrospective analysis of 230 women undergoing laparoscopic procedure without concomitant hysterectomy with transvaginal specimen extraction via posterior colpotomy. There were no cases of postoperative dyspareunia reported. Out of 6.5% complications recorded during the study, only one (0.1%) adverse event was related to colpotomy; that was bleeding from vaginal angle.[6]

Paradoxically, although the transvaginal route is being used increasingly by nongynecological surgeons during conventional or natural orifice transluminal endoscopic surgery (NOTES), most gynecologist are reluctant to perform vaginal colpotomy. The possible concerns may be due to risk of postoperative dyspareunia, pelvic infections, surgical damage to rectum or vaginal dehiscence or impact on future childbearing.

We should learn the art of vaginal surgery from our senior and eminent teachers. The vaginal route represents by definition one of the most logical and accessible ways to enter the pelvic cavity for gynecologists. We should be availing the advantages of the natural orifice extraction procedure for gynecological surgeries even in the presence of benign adnexal pathology.

REFERENCES

1. Maresh MJ, Metcalf MA, Mcpherson K, et al. The VALUE national hysterectomy study: description of the patient and their surgery. BJOG. 2002;109(3):302-12.
2. Dr Shirish Seth has performed vaginal oopherctomy in 1500 women, with a failure rate of 3-4%.
3. Sheth SS. The place of oophorectomy at vaginal hysterectomy. Br J Obstet Gynecol. 1991;98(7):662-6.
4. Sheth S, Malpani A. Routine prophylactic oopherectomy at the time of vaginal hysterectomy in postmenopausal women. Arch Gynecol Obstet. 1992;251(2):87-91.
5. Sheth S. Adnexactomy for benign pathology at vaginal hysterectomy without laparoscopic assistance. BJOG. 2002;109:1401-5.
6. Uccella S, Cromi A, Bogani G, et al. Transvaginal specimen extraction at laparoscopy without concomitant hysterectomy: our experience and systematic review of literature. J Minim Invasive Gynecol. 2013;20(5):583-90.

Chapter 5

Nondescent Vaginal Hysterectomy in Previous Lower Segment Cesarean Section

RM Saraogi

"Our doubts are traitors and make us lose the good we oft might win by fearing to attempt."

William Shakespeare

INTRODUCTION

Nondescent vaginal hysterectomy (NDVH) is removal of uterus through vagina in absence of descent. Vaginal route is preferred for removing uteri as it gives natural route, is scarless, and gives safer results than abdominal route in terms of complications. Langenbeck first performed vaginal hysterectomy in 1813. NDVH was pioneered by Haene Y in 1934. Because of increased cesarean sections, women undergoing hysterectomies with cesarean sections are increasing. Earlier previous cesarean section was relative contraindication to vaginal hysterectomy due to uterovesical adhesions and risk for unintended cystostomy. Skill and experience of surgeon is important in determining approach route. In older days, the vaginal hysterectomy was limited only for the prolapsed uterus but because of improved obstetric practice there is reduced incidence and severity of the genital prolapse. So it is now time for the gynecologist to master the vaginal route for the removal of nondescended uterus as hysterectomy can be brought to the level of relatively safe and simple operation. In modern India, S Sheth has brought forth new dimension in NDVH with his experience of 5,655 vaginal hysterectomies.[1]

Nondescent vaginal hysterectomy is safe, less invasive technique with benefits of shorter hospital stay and faster recovery. It is surgical method of choice for benign conditions of uterus and should be a primary method for removal of uterus, if not contraindicated. The criteria for NDVH are uterine size not more than 16 weeks (by clinical judgment) with normal uterine mobility. Exclusion criteria are nonmobile uterus, any malignancy, and adnexal masses.

In all cases, a per vaginum examination should be done under anesthesia before starting the surgery to again have an idea about size, mobility of uterus, and any adnexal mass. Cervicofundal sign by Dr Shirish Sheth to see for dimpling implying that there were dense adhesions with the anterior abdominal wall, such cases are better done by laparoscopic assisted vaginal hysterectomy (LAVH).

A major factor in determining the route of hysterectomy is transvaginal accessibility of the uterus.[2] Two factors limit accessibility, an undescended, immobile uterus and a vagina narrower than two finger breadths, especially at the apex. Determining whether the pathology is confined to or extends beyond the confines of the uterus is critical to selecting the most appropriate route of hysterectomy. The presence of severe endometriosis, adnexal pathology, and adhesions because of previous pelvic surgeries contraindicate vaginal hysterectomy.

TECHNIQUE (FIGS. 1A TO K)

- Anesthesia: Spinal-epidural
- Position: Dorsal lithotomy
- Draping and painting with betadine
- Labial sutures and bladder catheterization as usual
- Posterior cul-de-sac can be opened first

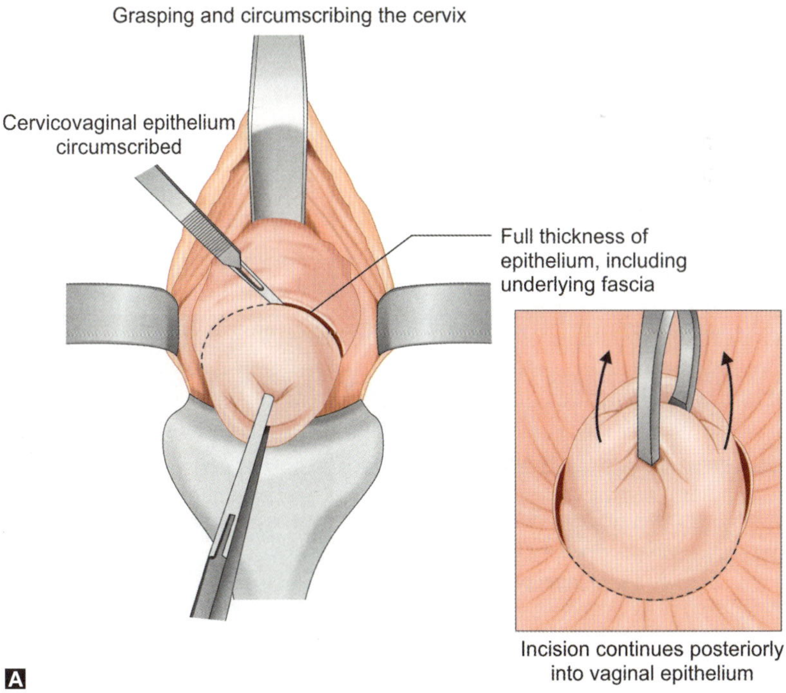

Fig. 1A:

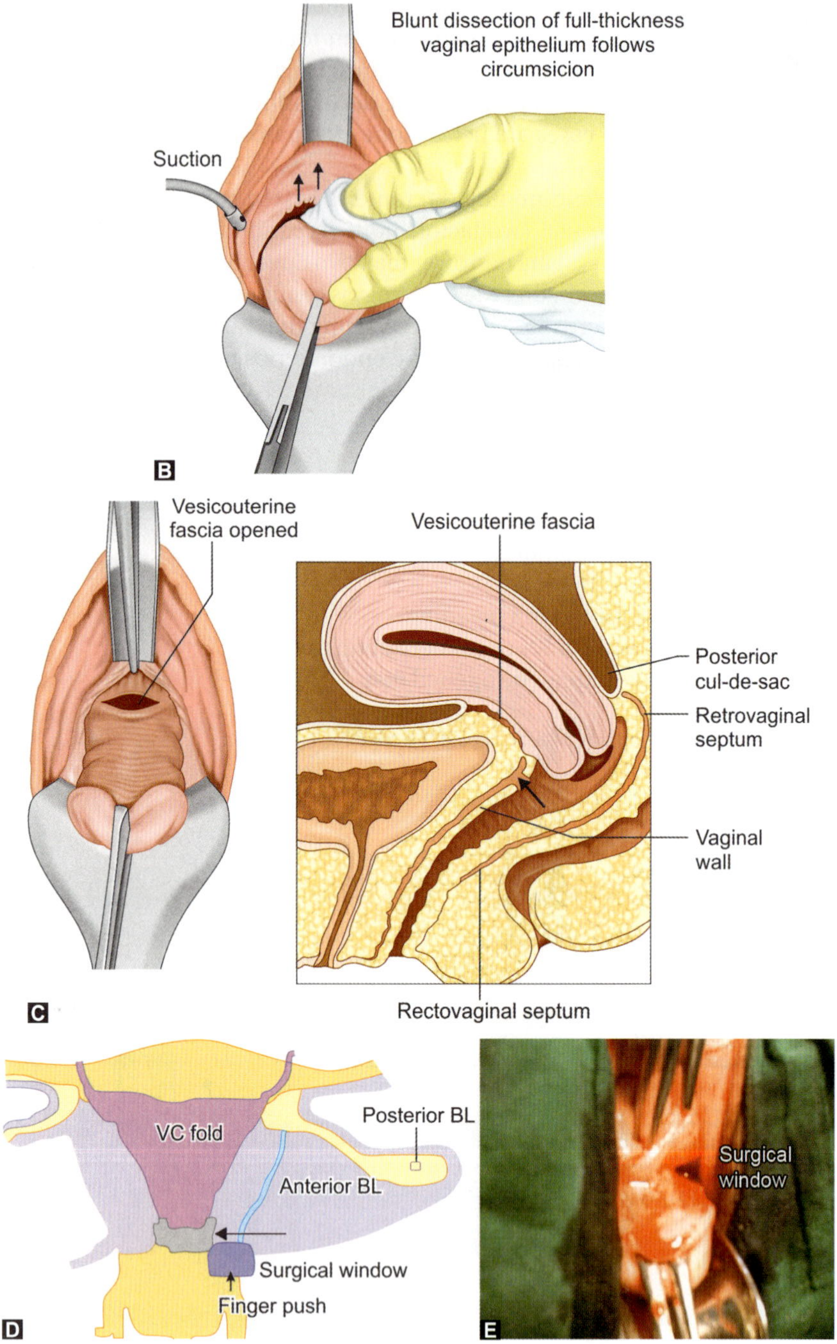
Blunt dissection of full-thickness vaginal epithelium follows circumsicion
Suction
B
Vesicouterine fascia opened
Vesicouterine fascia
Posterior cul-de-sac
Retrovaginal septum
Vaginal wall
Rectovaginal septum
C
VC fold
Posterior BL
Anterior BL
Surgical window
Finger push
D
Surgical window
E

Figs. 1B to E:

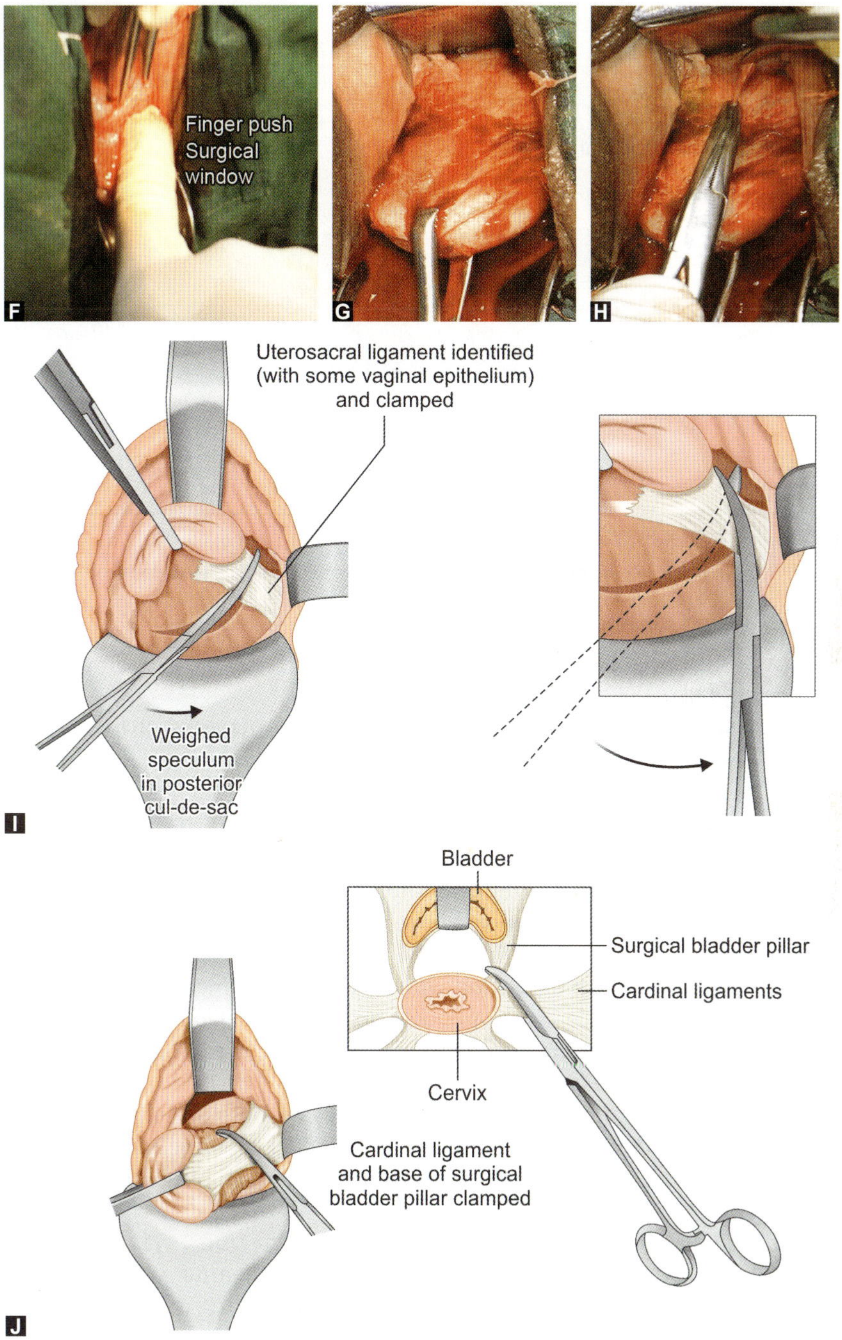
Finger push
Surgical
window
F
G
H
Uterosacral ligament identified
(with some vaginal epithelium)
and clamped
Weighed
speculum
in posterior
cul-de-sac
I
Bladder
Surgical bladder pillar
Cardinal ligaments
Cervix
Cardinal ligament
and base of surgical
bladder pillar clamped
J

Figs. 1F to J:

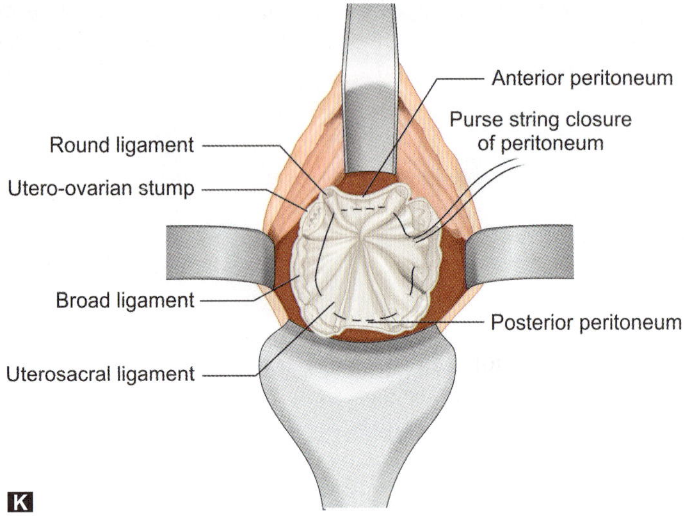

Fig. 1K:

Figs. 1A to K: Technique of performing nondescent vaginal hysterectomy.

- Anterior cul-de-sac:
  - Bladder separated with sharp dissection
  - Mayo curved scissors tips are pointed downward (30° angle to the plane of the cervix)
  - Lateral window may be used.

Try to push finger laterally on the cervix. There is a loose covering tissue leads to broad ligament. This is called surgical window. As a rule bladder is nonadherent and free in its lateral one-fifth. Use this window to enter over the anterior surface of broad ligament. Once you enter the broad ligament, come medially by hooking the index finger. Then we will see vesicocervical ligament. Cut the tissues by sharp dissection with scissor under finger protection and you will be in right space to see vesicocervical peritoneal fold.

Uterosacral and cardinal ligaments are clamped, cut, and ligated. Bilateral clamping of uterine vessels is done.

After clamping and ligating uterine arteries on both sides, if the size of uterus is big then debulking techniques like bisection, decoring, myomectomy, or a combination of these methods are done to facilitate vaginal delivery of uterus.

After delivering the uterus in the vagina, hysterectomy was completed by applying bilateral cornual clamps, cutting, and ligating it properly. All the pedicles were rechecked for any bleeding or oozing and vault closed meticulously.

For moderate to large sized uteri with benign conditions, techniques like bisection, coring, and morcellation may be adopted in an attempt to reduce the uterine volume prior to removal. Advantages of doing NDVH over abdominal hysterectomy are due to no scar, no adhesions, no hernia, no wound gap, associated urogynecological procedures can also be performed, less operative time, less blood loss, less anesthetics complications, largely extraperitoneal dissection to prevent injury to bowel, bladder and ureter, minimal bowel handling, no paralytic ileus, shorter hospital stay, fast recovery, low cost, less thromboembolic phenomena, less mortality and morbidity, natural, and simple route for drainage. Urinary tract injury is also less common in NDVH than other routes. Nowadays fibroid up to 16 weeks size and adnexal pathology can be also removed by vaginally. In high-risk patients NDVH is a preferred method for removal of uterus.

Vaginal hysterectomy in women with nondescent and moderately enlarged uteri is safe. A combination of morcellation techniques is often needed and the surgeon needs to be familiar with them. With experience, operative time, blood loss, and complications can be reduced considerably. Thus this scarless approach should be chosen as a preferred method of hysterectomy and a previous scar should not be a deterrent.

REFERENCES

1. Sheth SS. The scope of vaginal hysterectomy. Eur J Obstet Gynecol Reprod Biol. 2004;115(2):224-30.
2. Kovac SR, Barhan S, Lister M, et al. Guidelines for the selection of the route of hysterectomy: application in a resident clinic population. Am J Obstet Gynecol. 2002;187(6):1521-7.

Chapter 6

Vault Prolapse

Haresh U Doshi

INTRODUCTION

Vault prolapse is defined as the descent of vaginal vault below a point 2 cm less than the total vaginal length above the plane of hymen.

INCIDENCE

Reported incidence varies from 2% to 43%.[1] It is 11.6% of hysterectomies performed for prolapse and 1.8% for other benign diseases.[2] Vaginal vault **prolapse** can occur in patients months or years after a hysterectomy in conjunction with other pelvic floor defects such as cystocele, rectocele, or enterocele.

SYMPTOMS

They are variably present and like prolapse increase with time. These include:

- Protrusion or bulge from the vagina
- Pelvic pressure or pain
- Bleeding or vaginal discharge from ulceration
- Bladder and bowel symptoms: Difficulty in voiding or constipation. Some women need to elevate the prolapse to urinate or defecate
- Sexual dysfunction and/or dyspareunia.

The number of cases of vault prolapse are going to increase as longevity is increased with the improvement of quality of life in old age and growing interest in maintaining the capacity for sexual activity beyond the menopause.

ETIOLOGY

Preventable Factors

- *Hysterectomy:* Vault prolapse can occur after any hysterectomy if proper care is not taken to support the vaginal vault and obliterate the cul-de-sac. If we look at the different types of hysterectomies
  - Incidence least after total laparoscopic hysterectomy (TLH)
  - Incidence less after abdominal hysterectomy (AH)
  - Incidence more after nondescent vaginal hysterectomy (NDVH)
  - Incidence maximum after vaginal hysterectomy for prolapse (VH)
- Obstetric factors like multiparity and prolonged 2nd stage of labor
- Obesity
- Increased intra-abdominal pressure.

Nonpreventable Factors

- Aging—degenerative process and estrogen deficiency
- Race and ethnic factor
- Connective tissue disorder, neurological disorder, e.g. diabetes.

Elective cesarean section and timely episiotomy have been shown to decrease the incidence of prolapse. Cesarean section is a major surgery and cannot be recommended just for the prevention of future prolapse.

Royal College of Obstetricians and Gynaecologists (RCOG)/British Society of Urogynaecology (BSUG) Joint Guideline (Green-top guideline No. 46)[1] of 2015 for preventive techniques at hysterectomy states:

- McCall culdoplasty at the time of vaginal hysterectomy is effective in preventing posthysterectomy vault prolapse (PHVP). (Level B)
- Suturing the cardinal and uterosacral ligaments to the vaginal cuff at the time of hysterectomy is effective in preventing PHVP following both abdominal and vaginal hysterectomies. (Level B)
- Sacrospinous fixation (SSF) at the time of vaginal hysterectomy should be considered when the vault descends to the introitus during closure. (Level C)
- Subtotal hysterectomy is not recommended for the prevention of PHVP. (Level A)

American Association of Gynecologic Laparoscopists (AAGL) Practice Guidelines 2014[3] on the prevention of apical prolapse at the time of benign hysterectomy states:

- McCall's culdoplasty may be performed at the time of vaginal hysterectomy for nonprolapse related disease to reduce the risk of PHVP for up to 3 years (Level B)
- Uterosacral ligament suspension may be performed at the time of abdominal (Level B) and laparoscopic (Level C) hysterectomy to reduce the risk of PHVP

- Sacrospinous ligament fixation and abdominal sacral colpopexy are not recommended for the prevention of prolapse at the time of hysterectomy for nonprolapse related disease (Level C).

PREVENTION OF VAULT PROLAPSE

The prevention of vault prolapse at hysterectomy is:

- *Vault support:* These procedures are either vaginal or abdominal.
  - Vaginal procedures
    - Sacrospinous fixation
    - High uterosacral ligament suspension
    - Iliococcygeus fixation
  - Abdominal procedures
    - Colposacropexy
    - Uterosacral suspension
- *Enterocoele repair:* This can be done at vaginal or abdominal hysterectomy.
  - Vaginal route:
    - McCall's culdoplasty
      - Internal culdoplasty
      - External culdoplasty
      - Modified culdoplasty
  - Abdominal route:
    - Moschowitz suture
    - Halban's suture.

Many surgeries mentioned under prevention above are also the standard surgeries for treatment.

TREATMENT OF VAULT PROLAPSE

Nonsurgical

They are palliative treatment. These include pessary and Kegel exercise. Innert silicone pessary is useful in very old frail patients, medically ill unfit patients and patients not willing for surgery. Kegel exercise may be useful in mildly symptomatic cases. It increases the muscle tone and limits the progression of disease and may alleviate the symptoms.

Surgical

Different procedures have been suggested.

These can be reconstructive or obliterative. Reconstructive surgeries can be performed either vaginally or abdominally.

Abdominal procedures can be performed by conventional laparotomy or by minimally invasive techniques, including laparoscopy and robotic-assisted laparoscopy.

Principles of Reconstructive Surgical Treatment

- Discuss various routes and options with the patient with pros and cons
- Consider patient factors such as age, comorbid conditions and pelvic pathology if any
- Avoid distortion of vaginal axis
- Preserve adequate vaginal length (≥ 7 cm) as well as normal vaginal caliber
- Correct all defects
- Choose most appropriate surgery for the patient.

"Let surgery fit to the patient rather than patient fit to surgery."

Vaginal procedures:

- Sacrospinous fixation
- McCall culdoplasty
- Iliococcygeus fixation
- Uterosacral suspension
- Posterior intravaginal slingoplasty

Abdominal procedures:

- Colposacropexy
- High uterosacral ligament suspension
- William Richardson's operation.

Two commonly performed surgeries are described here:

1. *Colposacropexy:* Gold standard for the treatment vault prolapse. 2 cm wide strips from anterior rectus sheath or merlex mesh is used to suspend the vaginal vault to the anterior sacral ligament in front of the third sacral vertebra. It can be done by open method or laparoscopically or robotic surgery (Fig. 1).

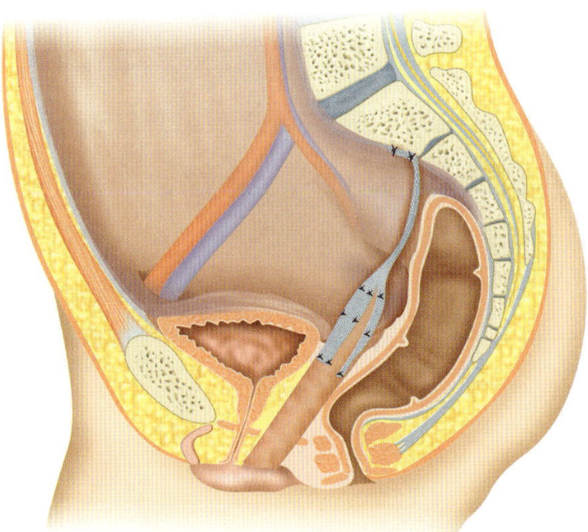

Fig. 1: Colposacropexy.

Advantages:
- High cure rate
- Dyspareunia less
- Can be done in short vagina
- More anatomical.

Disadvantages:
- Need more time
- More expertise
- Higher cost
- Higher postoperative morbidity.

2. *Sacrospinous fixation:* This procedure suspends the vault to the sacrospinous ligament. The ligament is commonly approached by posterior vaginal route. Sutures are placed on the sacrospinous ligament by ligament carrier or hook and are secured to the vaginal vault. Generally done unilaterally and on right side since the bowel enters the rectum on the left side. Doing it bilaterally is not found superior (Fig. 2).

   Success rate of SSF has been quoted to vary from 67% to 94 % in several case series in different studies.

   Advantages:
   - Extraperitoneal
   - Not difficult to perform
   - Low postoperative morbidity
   - Associated anterior and posterior vaginal wall.

   Disadvantages:
   - Relatively high failure rate
   - Difficult to do in short vagina
   - Unilateral vaginal deflection
   - Occasionally nerve injuries and defects can be repaired vessel injuries.

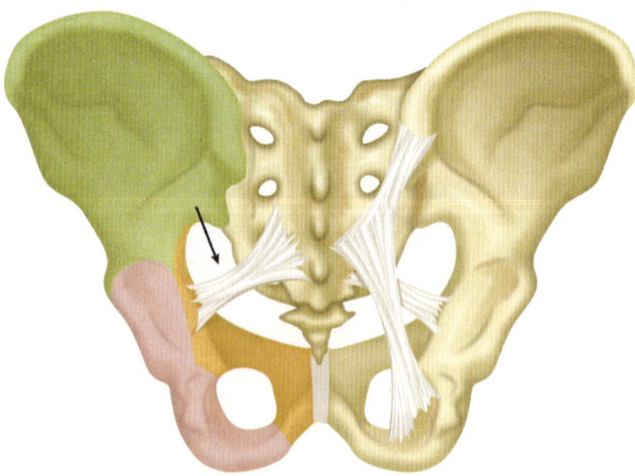

Fig. 2: Sacrospinous fixation.

Maher et al. (ACOG, 2004)[4] compared both the procedures by randomized prospective study and concluded that:

- Both the procedures are equally effective on long-term follow-up
- Sacrospinous fixation is better if posterior wall prolapse is predominant
- Abdominal sacropexy is better when anterior vaginal wall prolapse is predominant.

Use of mesh vaginally is not recommended for prevention of vault prolapse. Mesh cause erosion, infection and dyspareunia in many cases and Food and Drug Administration (FDA) has put it in high-risk category (Category III) device and restricted its use since 2011 for treatment of prolapse.[5]

Obliterative Procedures

Le Fort's colpocleisis is recommended when coital function is not required. Quadrilateral flaps from anterior and posterior vaginal walls are removed, and raw areas are sutured together. Goodall-power modification is practiced when coital function is required. Total colpocleisis on the other hand involves removal of all vaginal epithelium and suturing it together. There are up to 30% chances of postoperative stress urinary incontinence (SUI). Introital stitch as treatment is very rarely indicated.

CONCLUSION

- Suspension of vault at any method of hysterectomy is of prime importance
- Enterocoele repair at primary surgery is must
- McCall culdoplasty, colposacropexy and sacrospinous fixation are the best treatment options.

"In preparing for prolapse surgery the patient should have an understanding of the expected results *and* the surgeon should have understanding of the patient's expectations."

—William's Gynecology

REFERENCES

1. Posthysterectomy vaginal vault prolapse. Green-top Guideline No. 46. RCOG/BUSG joint guideline July 2015
2. Marchionni M, Bracco GL, Checcucci V, et al. True incidence of vaginal vault prolapse. thirteen years of experience. J Reprod Med. 1999;44:679-84.
3. AAGL Advancing Minimally Invasive Gynecology Worldwide. AAGL Practice Report: Practice Guidelines on the Prevention of Apical Prolapse at the Time of Benign Hysterectomy. J Minim Invasive Gynecol. 2014;21(5):715-22.
4. Maher CF, Qatawneh AM, Dwyer PL, et al. Abdominal sacral colpopexy or vaginal sacrospinous colpopexy for vaginal vault prolapse: a prospective randomized study. Am J Obstet Gynecol. 2004;190(1):20-6.
5. US Food and Drug Administration. FDA strengthens requirements for surgical mesh for the transvaginal repair of pelvic organ prolapse to address safety risks. Silver Spring: FDA; 2016.

Chapter 7

Vesicovaginal Fistula

Meenakshi Patel

INTRODUCTION

Vesicovaginal fistula (VVF) is the most common acquired fistula of urinary tract. Early attempts at repair met with little success. In 1852, Sims published his method for surgical treatment of VVF using transvaginal approach followed by Trendelenburg in 1888 who performed transabdominal VVF repair. It represents significant morbidity in female urology. Continuous wetness, bad odor, discomfort cause serious social problem. Successful repair of fistulas requires accurate diagnosis, timely repair using procedures with basic surgical principles and application of interposition flaps method of closure. Results depend on surgical skill and experience. Main complication is recurrence.

INCIDENCE

0.8/1,000 of all hysterectomy is complicated with VVF.

DEFINITION

Abnormal communication between bladder and vagina that allows continuous involuntary discharge of urine in to vaginal vault.

ETIOLOGY

It can be

- Congenital: Very rear

- Traumatic
  - Obstetric trauma: Direct injury to bladder wall by sharp instrument
    - Necrotic fistula: Develops within 5–7 days after labor, or surgery
    - Obstructive fistula
  - Surgical trauma
  - Direct trauma
- Inflammatory disease
- Malignant neoplasm
- Radiation necrosis.

SYMPTOMS

Incontinence of urine, lower abdominal pain, symptoms of vulvitis—cystitis.

HOW TO EVALUATE VESICOVAGINAL FISTULA

Evaluate the fistula by identifying size, site, type, number, scarring, recurrence, involvement of ureteric orifice, and involvement of sphincteric mechanism. *Prognosis depends on these.* Bigger the size more is complicated and more scarring—worst outcome. Small (0.5–1.5 cm) Medium (1.5–3 cm) Large (>3 cm): these usually involve loss of most of the anterior vaginal wall and a circumferential loss of the uterovesical (UV) junction.

Per vaginal (P/V): During palpation of anterior vaginal wall large fistula felt. Small fistula not felt.

P/S: Small and high fistula.

Dye test: Methylene blue on Sim's speculum.

Radiological: Computed tomography intravenous pyelogram (CT-IVP) and chromocystoscopy. Cystoscopy is done to determine the site, number and involvement of ureteric orifice.

MANAGEMENT

Medical Therapy

Transurethral/suprapubic catheter should be placed for 30 days. Estrogen therapy 4–6 weeks. Fistula less than 1 cm may resolve or decrease in size. Traumatic fistula heals within 30 days. But due to radiation, it will take longer time.

When to repair fistula: Repair for traumatic fistula within 8–12 weeks. Radiation fistula at the end of 1 year because of full resolution of tissue necrosis. Very few fistulas are repaired within 72 hours of original surgery. When tissues blood supply is normal.

Techniques of VVF repair:

- Vaginal approach: Latzko repair

- Abdominal approach
- Electrocautery
- Fibrin glue
- Endoscopic closure with fibrin glue
- Laparoscopic approach
- Using interposition grafts.

General Surgical Principle for Fistula Repair

- Proper diagnosis
- Adequate exposure of operative field to avoid inadvertent organ injury
- Homeostasis
- Mobilization of tissue
- Tissue closure under no tension. Take vaginal mucosa wall with pubovesical cervical fascia by interrupted stitches
- Water tight closure of bladder
- To avoid infection and inflammation of tissue
- Adequate blood supply at area of repair
- Continuous catheter drainage.

Preoperative Care

Antibiotic prophylaxis, treat vulvitis, renal function test, urine culture/sensitivity (C/S).

Vaginal Approach

Flap splitting operation—fistula tract is initially dilated with metal sound and insert small catheter it can be used as retractor during dissection. Saline is injected into the anterior vaginal wall around fistulous tract. An inverted J-shaped incision that circumscribes the fistula tract is made with long end of J extending to the apex of vagina. Circular incision around fistula. Two short longitudinal cuts upward and downward. Free mobilization of vaginal flaps from bladder over a wide area 1.5 cm around the fistula. The hole in bladder is closed by two layers of interrupted sutures. Nonabsorbable sutures should never be used, because a stone may form in the bladder later. 2/0, 3/0 Vicryl half-circle 25 mm round-bodied needles. Vagina is closed by interrupted sutures.

Advantages of vaginal approach:

- Minimal blood loss
- Low postoperative morbidity
- Short operative time and recovery time
- It obviates bowel manipulation, reducing operative morbidity in radiation associated VVF.

Contraindication of vaginal approach:

- Severely indurated vaginal epithelium around fistula
- Small capacity, poorly complaint bladder
- Repair requires ureteric reimplantation
- Involvement of other pelvic structure
- Vaginal stenosis.

Absolute Indication for Abdominal Approach

- Need for concomitant abdominal surgery
- Inability to expose the fistula vaginally
- Complex VVF involving ureter, ureteric orifice, and bowel.

Transabdominal O'Connor's Operation for Supratrigonal Fistula

Utilizes suprapubic area for extraperitoneal dissection of retropubic space to dissect the bladder and followed by large sagittal cystotomy until fistula reached. Fistulous tract is excised and two layers suturing closure. After omentum transposition between bladder and vaginal wall. Success rate 85–100%. Laparoscopic repair can be done with same steps.

Sim's Saucerization Operation

If tissues are too adherent and fibroses to do flap splitting. After failure of flap splitting, then technique is used. Edge of fistula excised removing a wider part of vaginal than of muscle wall of bladder. Edges of both organs are simultaneously coapted together by use of nonabsorbable sutures. Certain high fistulas are better treated by abdominal repair.

Modern Technique

Extravesical transperitoneal technique: Beneficial, when bladder is densely adherent to underlying tissues structures, endopelvic fascia. Use of peritoneal and omental grafts in large fistulas and bladder mucosal grafts as larger as 4 cm used successfully. 100% success rate.

Postoperative Care

The main aim includes—patient must be dry, drinking, draining. If patient becomes wet then catheter will be blocked, there is leaking around catheter, and repair has broken down. Acidification of urine is present. Vitamin C 500 mg three times/day should be given. Catheter should be kept for 14 days. After the catheter is removed patient should be instructed to void urine every 2 hours/day, every 4 hours/night. Avoid over distension and disruption of suture line. Avoid sexual intercourse for 3 months. Avoid pregnancy for 1 year. Lower segment cesarean section (LSCS) for all future pregnancy.

COMPLICATION

Recurrence fistula formation, ureteric injury or obstruction, vaginal stenosis, reduced bladder capacity, lower urinary tract symptoms, recurrent fistula can be managed conservatively with prolonged catheterization.

CONCLUSION

Vesicovaginal fistula continuous to challenge even with experienced surgeons. If small and treated immediately after the antecedent event, conservative therapy with prolonged bladder drainage may be effective. Role of surgery can be performed successfully through vaginal/abdominal route. Role of interposition of graft at the both route is viewed positively and adjutant techniques are needed for complex fistula. Adherence to strict surgical principles for fistula repair will result in optimal cure rates and prevents the recurrence.

Chapter 8

Obstetric Anal Sphincter Injuries

Mohan A Gadam

COMPLETE PERINEAL TEAR

This topic will cover basics of all degrees of fresh perineal tears (Obstetric anal sphincter injuries or OASIS) with particular emphasis on 3rd and 4th degree perineal tears. Significance of iatrogenic 3rd and 4th degree perineal tears in modern obstetric practice is unimaginable as it carries a heavy burden of medicolegal suits and consumer litigations. Obstetricians all over the world remain in fear psychosis and thus are under constant stress due to such litigations.

Onus lies on them to prove that they took all the necessary steps to avoid such an injury and while managing such a case they strictly adhered to the prevailing guidelines and good practices. Needless to say that the documentation was in perfect order. One can avoid conviction, if one follows norms strictly as this is a known complication of any delivery.

For convenience, I would divide this topic in following three headings:

1. Basic anatomy of perineum
2. 3rd and 4th degree perineal tears or OASIS
3. Principles of surgical repair and related management options.

INTRODUCTION

- Out of total, 85% of women who have a vaginal birth have some form of perineal trauma
- The morbidity associated with perineal injury and repair is a major health problem.

PERINEAL TRAUMA

Trauma can be deliberate to widen the passage of outer birth canal or spontaneous while conducting a difficult vaginal delivery or an operative vaginal delivery (Flowchart 1).

ANATOMY OF PERINEUM

Just to recapitulate, following structures are usually cut while giving an episiotomy:

- Vaginal mucosa or skin
- Perineal skin
- Subcutaneous tissue and the Scarpa's fascia
- Muscles of superficial and deep perineal pouch and the fascia covering them
- Few blood vessels, lymphatics and the nerve terminals (Fig. 1).

Flowchart 1: Perineal trauma.

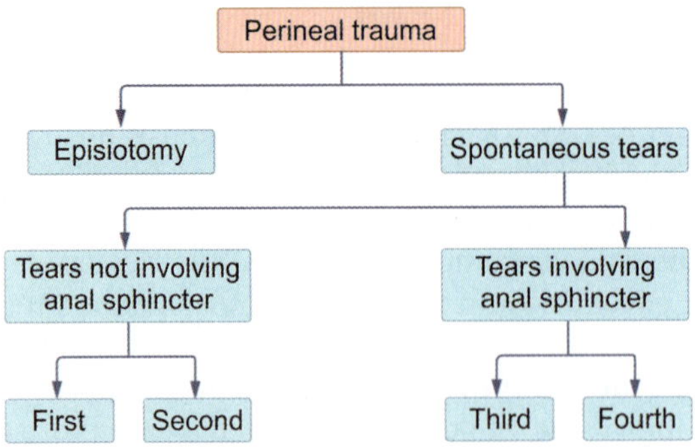

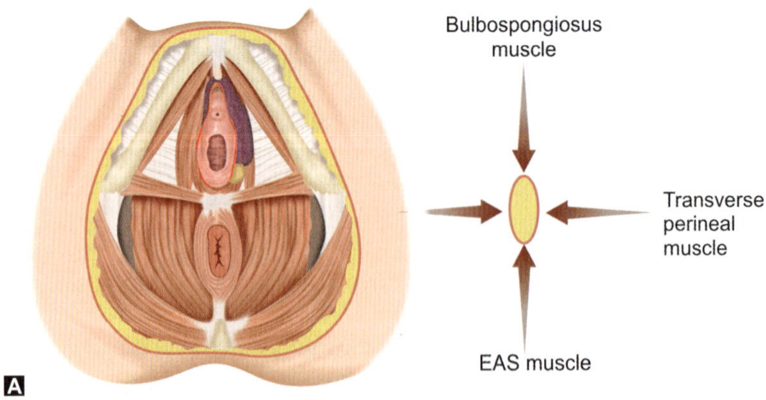

Fig. 1A:

(EAS: external anal sphincter)

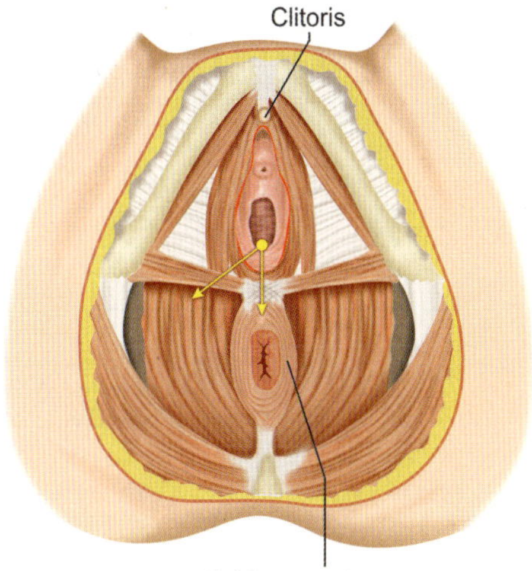

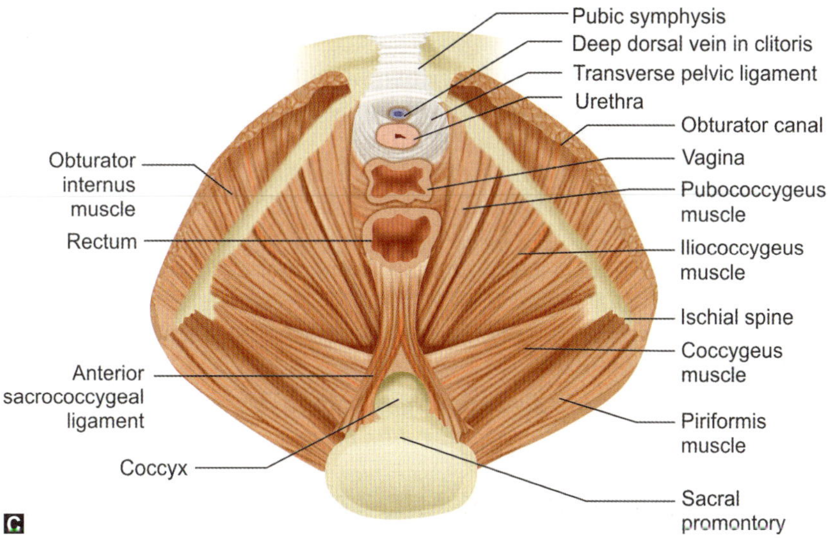

Figs. 1B and B:

Figs. 1A to C: Anatomy of perineum.

MECHANISM OF ANAL SPHINCTER INJURIES

Anal sphincter, being close to vaginal outlet and being part of superficial perineal pouch, is most vulnerable to any obstetric trauma. It expands almost 2.5 times its original size during parturition. During difficult spontaneous or an operative vaginal delivery, an episiotomy is likely to extend onto anal sphincter without any realization and often due to inadequate perineal support. At times, this can often be due to an episiotomy which is either not adequate to the situation or not in proper direction (Episiotomy should ideally start at fourchette and be mediolateral and should lie at an angle 30–60° as shown in Figure 2).

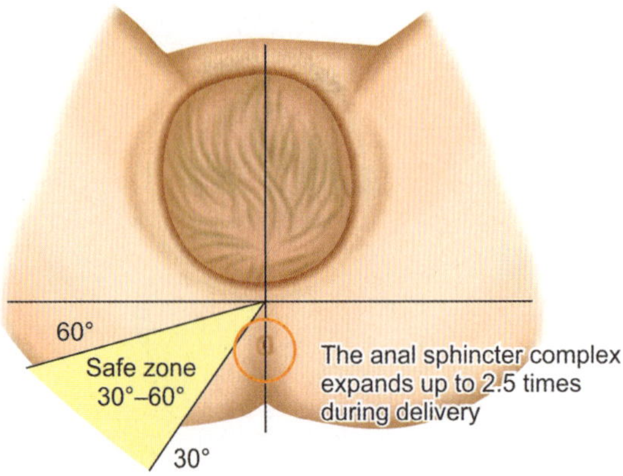

Fig. 2: Mechanism of anal sphincter injuries.

CLASSIFICATION OF PERINEAL TEARS

The following classification described by Sultan has been adopted by the International Consultation on Incontinence and the Royal College of Obstetricians and Gynaecologists (RCOG).

- *First degree:* Vaginal epithelium and perineal skin
- *Second degree:* Vaginal epithelium + perineal skin + perineal muscles
- *Third degree:* In addition to involvement of structures in second degree perineal tear, there is additional involvement of anal sphincter without anal mucosa being involved
- *Fourth degree:* Involvement of vaginal mucosa, perineal skin anal sphincter along with anal mucosa.

Note: If there is any doubt about the degree of third-degree tear, it is advisable to classify it to the higher degree rather than the lower degree.

CLASSIFICATION OF 3RD AND 4TH DEGREE PERINEAL INJURY

The RCOG guidelines further classify 3rd and 4th degree perineal injuries as (The following classification described by Sultan has been adopted by the International Consultation on Incontinence and the RCOG):

- 3rd degree: Anal sphincter tear
  - 3a = <50% external sphincter thickness
  - 3b = >50% external sphincter thickness
  - 3c = Internal sphincter torn
- 4th degree: Involvement of anal mucosa along with entire internal and external anal sphincter (EAS) (Fig. 3).

Note: If there is any doubt about the degree of 3rd degree tear, it is advisable to classify it to the higher degree rather than the lower degree.

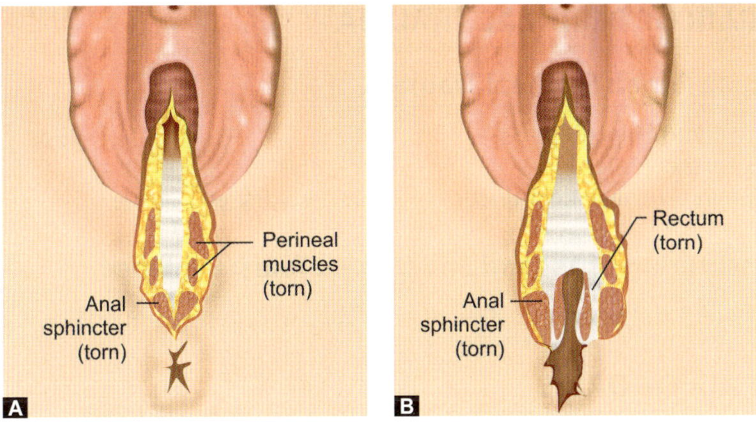

Figs. 3A and B: Perineal tears: (A) Third degree; and (B) Fourth degree.

PREDICTION AND PREVENTION

Obstetric Anal Sphincter Injury Prediction

Obstetric anal sphincter injury prediction can often be predicted:

- Clinicians need to be aware of the risk factors for OASIS
- Clinicians should be aware, however, that risk factors do not allow the accurate prediction of OASIS.

Can Obstetric Anal Sphincter Injury be Prevented?

- Clinicians should explain to women that the evidence for the protective effect of episiotomy is conflicting
- Mediolateral episiotomy should be considered in instrumental deliveries
- Where episiotomy is indicated, the mediolateral technique is recommended, with careful attention to ensure that the angle is 60° away from the midline when the perineum is distended
- Perineal protection at crowning can be protective
- Warm compression during the second stage of labor reduces the risk of OASIS.

IDENTIFICATION OF OBSTETRIC ANAL SPHINCTER INJURIES

How can the identification of OASIS be improved?

All women having a vaginal delivery are at risk of sustaining OASIS or isolated rectal button hole tears. They should, therefore, be examined systematically, including a digital rectal examination, to assess the severity of damage, particularly prior to suturing.

REPAIR OF PERINEAL TRAUMA

Why to Repair Perineal Trauma?

- To control bleeding
- To prevent infection
- To prevent anal incontinence in 3rd and 4th degree.

Nonsuturing of 1st and 2nd Degree Tears: Evidence

- 1st and 2nd degree: Unsutured associated with poorer wound healing.

REPAIR OF OASIS

General Principles

- Repair of 3rd and 4th degree tears should be conducted by an appropriately trained clinician or by a trainee under supervision
- Repair should take place in an operating theater, under regional or general anesthesia, with good lighting and with appropriate instruments
- If there is excessive bleeding, a vaginal pack should be inserted and the woman should be taken to the theater as soon as possible
- Figure-of-eight sutures should be avoided during the repair of OASIS because they are hemostatic in nature and may cause tissue ischemia
- A rectal examination should be performed after the repair to ensure that sutures have not been inadvertently inserted through the anorectal mucosa. If a suture is identified, it should be removed.

Repair of Perineal Trauma

- Suture materials
- Suture technique
- Adherence to basic principles of surgery
- Comprehensive postoperative management (Key to success).

Evidence for Suture Materials

Cochrane review:
Absorbable synthetic materials (synthetic delayed absorbable) versus Catgut.
Synthetic delayed absorbable sutures are associated with:
- ↓ Perineal pain
- ↓Analgesic use
- ↓Dehiscence wounds
- ↓ Resuturing.

Prerequisites Before Starting Perineal Repair

- Per vaginal and per rectal to check extent of perineal trauma

- Check instruments, suture pack, materials, adequate lighting
- Ensure that the wound is adequately anesthetized (10–20 mL lignocaine 1%)—do not inject local through the skin
- If needed, ensure that appropriate supervision or support is available prior to commencing the repair.

Instrument Trolley (Fig. 4)

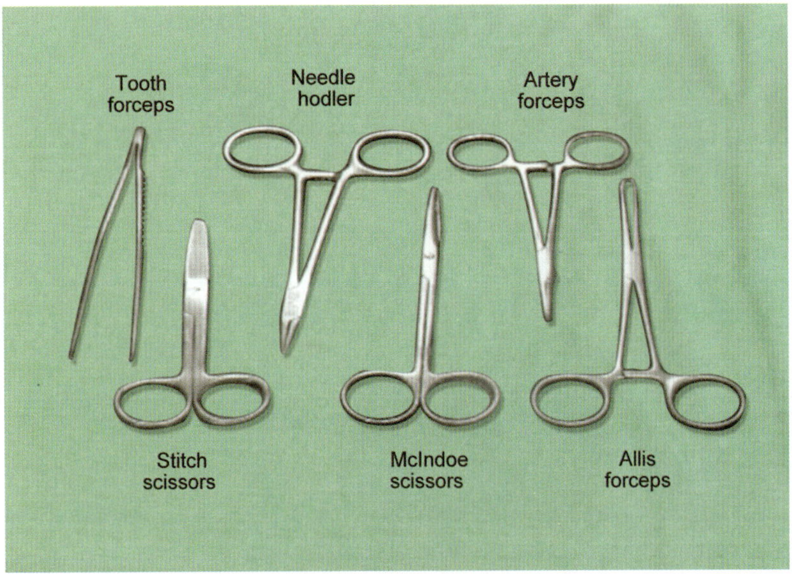

Fig. 4: Instruments.

STEPS

Step 1: Suturing the Vagina (Fig. 5)

- Identify the apex of the vaginal wound
- Close the vaginal skin with a loose continuous stitch
- At the fourchette, insert the needle through the skin to emerge in the center of the perineal trauma.

Step 2: Suturing the Muscle Layer (Fig. 6)

- Check the depth of the trauma—it may be necessary to insert two layers of sutures
- Close the perineal muscle with a continuous nonlocking stitch, taking care not to leave any dead space.

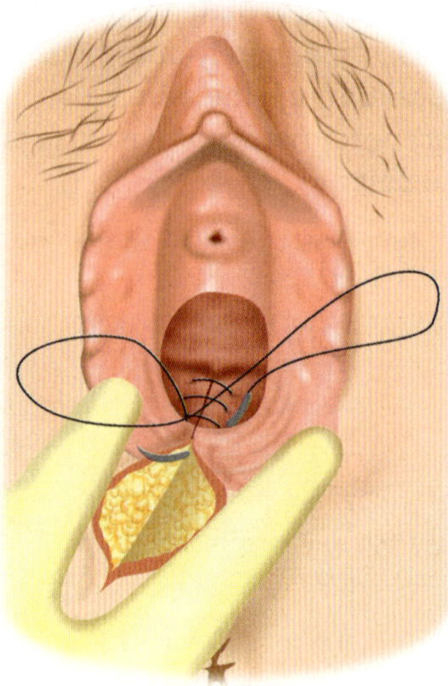

Fig. 5: Suturing the vagina.

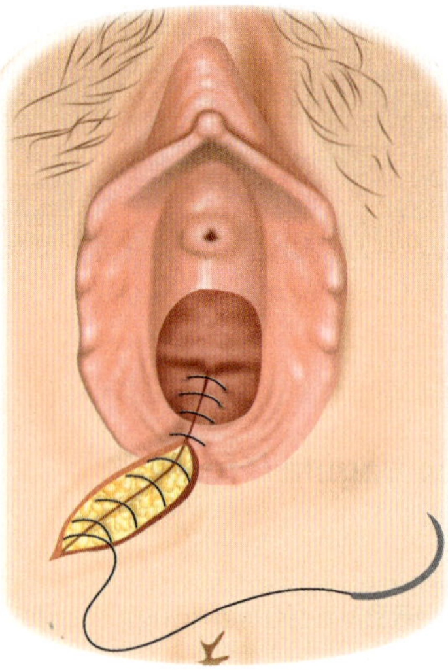

Fig. 6: Suturing the muscle layer.

Step 3: Suturing the Perineal Skin (Fig. 7)

- At the inferior end of the wound, bring the needle out under the skin surface
- Stitches placed below the skin surface in the subcutaneous layer, thus avoiding the profusion of nerve endings
- Take bites of tissue from each side of the wound until the hymenal remnants are reached
- Secure the finished repair with a loop knot tied in the vagina.

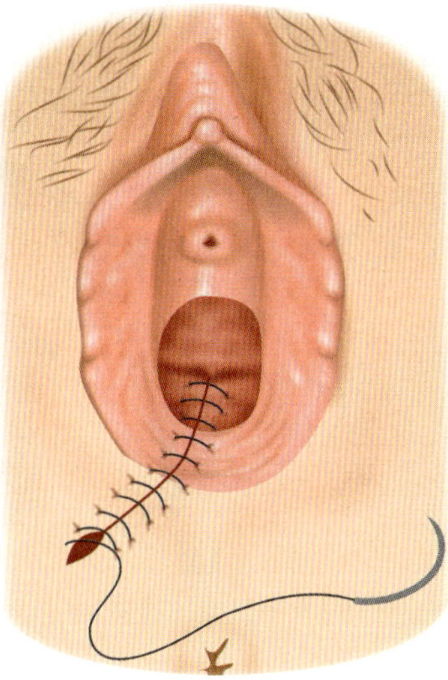

Fig. 7: Suturing the perineal skin.

RECOMMENDED MATERIAL AND TECHNIQUE FOR 1ST AND 2ND DEGREE TEARS OR EPISIOTOMY

There is level 1A evidence for use of (SDA) Rapide suture material for 1st and 2nd degree tears along with continuous nonlocking technique for all layers of perineal repair.

Rationale: Continuous Technique

- *No knots*: Sutures accommodate themselves to swelling as it occurs
- Tight sutures cause pain especially if the wound becomes edematous; may cause tissue hypoxia and delay healing
- Skin sutures inserted into subcutaneous layer thus avoiding nerve endings in skin surface giving rise to less pain
- *Economical*: Single suture used.

SUTURING OF 3RD AND 4TH DEGREE PERINEAL TEARS

Which techniques should be used to accomplish the repair of the anorectal mucosa?

The torn anorectal mucosa should be repaired with sutures using either the continuous or interrupted technique. The knots should lie in anal canal.

Which techniques should be used to accomplish the repair of the internal anal sphincter?

Where the torn internal anal sphincter (IAS) can be identified, it is advisable to repair this separately with interrupted or mattress sutures without any attempt to overlap the IAS.

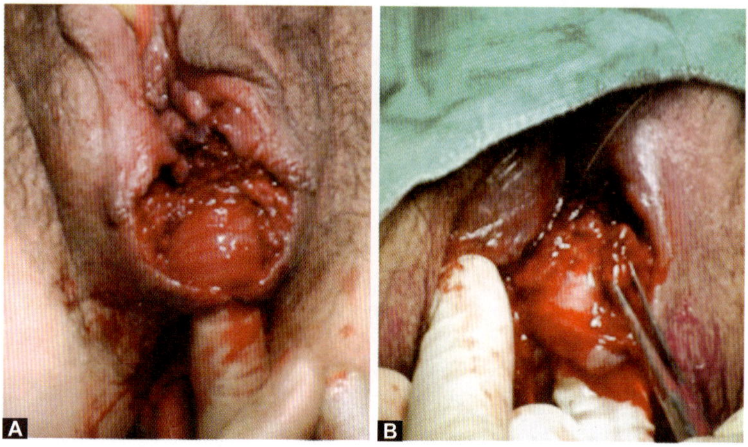

Figs. 8A and B: Repair of anal sphincters.

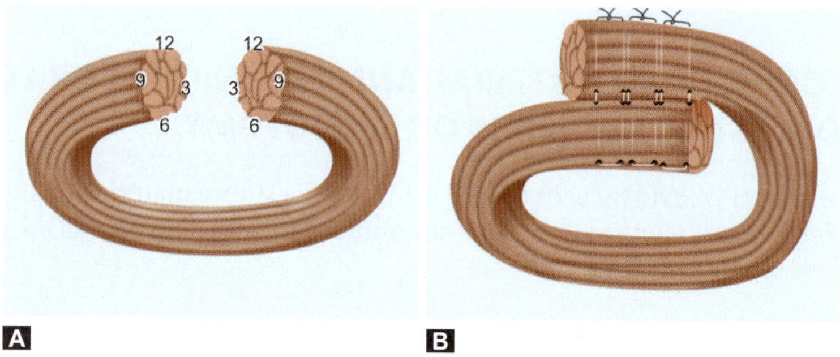

Figs. 9A and B: Techniques to repair the external anal sphincter. (A) End-to-end (approximation) method; (B) Overlap technique.

Which techniques should be used to repair the external anal sphincter?

- For repair of a full thickness EAS tear, either an overlapping or an end-to-end (approximation) method can be used with equivalent outcomes
- For partial thickness (all 3a and some 3b) tears, an end-to-end technique should be used (Figs. 8 and 9).

CHOICE OF SUTURE MATERIALS

Which suture materials should be used to accomplish repair of OASIS?

- 3-0 polyglactin should be used to repair the anorectal mucosa as it may cause less irritation and discomfort than polydioxanone (PDS) sutures
- When repair of the EAS and/or IAS muscle is being performed, either monofilament sutures such as 3-0 PDS or modern braided sutures such as 2-0 polyglactin can be used with equivalent outcomes

- When obstetric anal sphincter repairs are being performed, the burying of surgical knots beneath the superficial perineal muscles is recommended to minimize the risk of knot and suture migration to the skin.

END-TO-END (APPROXIMATION) METHOD

Sphincter Identification (Figs. 10A to D)

- Basic principles
- Difficult trauma: Experienced operator
  - OT
  - GA/RA
- Indwelling catheter 24 hours
- Ensure good anatomical alignment: Hemostasis, asepsis and anatomical closure are the key to the success
- Rectal examination at the end.

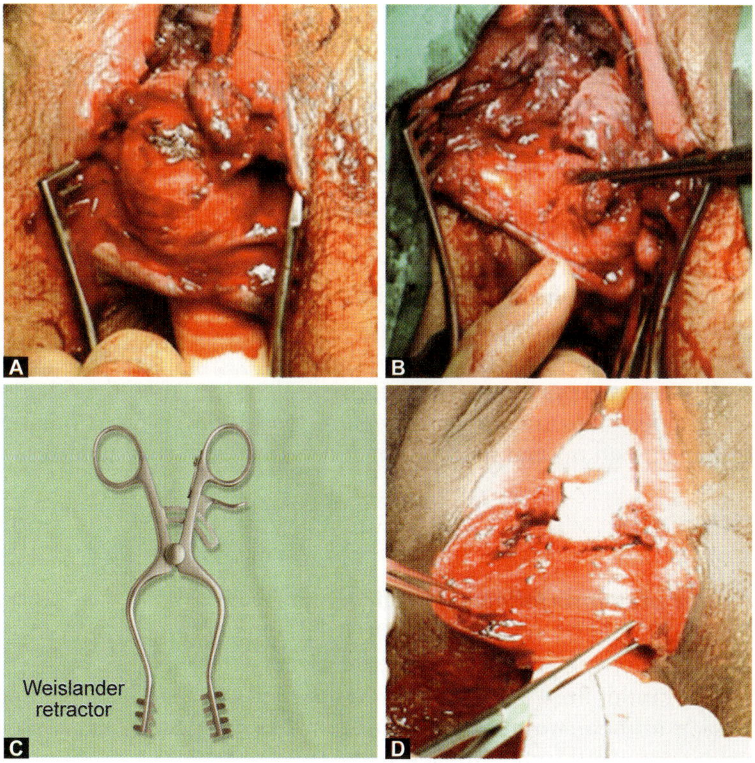

Figs. 10A to D: Sphincter identification.

Finally

- Check the finished repair is anatomically correct
- No bleeding
- Per vaginal—insert two fingers
- Per rectal
- Check swabs and instruments
- Document
- Pain relief
- Discuss diet, hygiene, pelvic floor exercises.

POSTOPERATIVE CARE

- Adequate appropriate broad spectrum antibiotics (Cefuroxime 1500 mg and metronidazole 500 mg) intravenous intraoperatively
- Continued orally: 1 week
- Stool softeners
- Soft or full diet from day one
- Pelvic floor exercise for 6–12 weeks following repair.

FOLLOW-UP

- Review—6–12 weeks
- Symptomatic—endoanal ultrasonography and anorectal manometry
- Advisable to follow-up for at least 12 months.

RECOMMENDED PRACTICE

- Rectal examination after every delivery
- Classify the perineal injuries accurately
- Analgesia or anesthesia as appropriate
- Evidence-based practice—use of appropriate materials and methods
- Trained person to undertake the repair—recognition of own limitations
- Training programs and supervision of perineal repairs for all levels.

PROGNOSIS

What is the prognosis following surgical repair?

- Women should be advised that 60–80% of women are asymptomatic 12 months following delivery and EAS repair
- Several randomized controlled studies carried out since 2000 comparing overlap and end-to-end techniques of EAS repair have reported low incidences of anal incontinence symptoms in both arms, with 60–80% of women described as asymptomatic at 12 months.

FUTURE DELIVERIES

What advice should women be given following an obstetric anal sphincter injury concerning future pregnancies and mode of delivery?

- All women who sustained OASIS in a previous pregnancy should be counseled about the mode of delivery and this should be clearly documented in the notes
- The role of prophylactic episiotomy in subsequent pregnancies is not known and therefore an episiotomy should only be performed if clinically indicated
- All women who have sustained OASIS in a previous pregnancy and who are symptomatic have abnormal endovaginal ultrasonography and/or manometry should be counseled regarding the option of elective cesarean birth
- There were no systematic reviews or randomized controlled trials to suggest the best method of delivery following OASIS. The risk of sustaining a further 3rd and 4th degree tear after a subsequent delivery is 5–7%
- The risks of a subsequent vaginal delivery after a 3rd degree tear have been assessed, with 17% of women developing worsening fecal symptoms after a second vaginal delivery. This seemed to occur if there had been fecal incontinence beyond 3 months but resolution by 6 months after the index delivery
- There are no studies to suggest that prophylactic episiotomy in the subsequent delivery would prevent OASIS. Hence, the decision to perform an episiotomy during the subsequent delivery after previous OASIS needs to be a clinical decision independent of the previous OASIS
- If the woman is symptomatic or shows abnormally low anorectal manometric pressures and/or endoanal ultrasonographic defects, an elective cesarean section may be considered
- One prospective study of pregnant women who previously sustained OASIS evaluated a protocol in which women who had a sonographic defect of the external sphincter of more than 30° accompanied by an incremental squeeze pressure of less than 20 mm Hg were offered a cesarean section. All other women were advised to have a vaginal delivery. Short-term follow-up of this cohort of 73 women showed that the women who underwent vaginal delivery suffered no significant deterioration in anal sphincter function or quality of life
- Units should have a clear protocol for the management of OASIS
- Documentation of the anatomical structures involved, the method of repair and the suture materials should be made. The woman should be fully informed about the nature of her tear and the offer of follow-up should be made, all supported by relevant written information
- At present, the occurrence of OASIS is not considered substandard care because it is a known complication of vaginal delivery

- However, failure to recognize anal sphincter damage or carry out an adequate repair may be considered substandard care
- A poor technique, poor selection of materials or poor healing may cause a repair to fail
- Clear documentation, preferably using a drawing, together with providing the woman with an explanation and patient information leaflet, is important.

"Let us end here with a very well-quoted sentence from Bailey and Love's short textbook on surgery: If you do not put your finger in it, you might put your foot in it."

Chapter 9

Colpocleisis or Le Fort Operation for Prolapse

Ramesh Desale

INTRODUCTION

Le fort first described a new method for the cure of prolapsed in 1877. The Le fort partial colpocleisis (Fig. 1) is an obliterative vaginal procedure that approximates anterior and posterior vaginal walls. This surgery effectively replaces the prolapsed vaginal vaults into abdominal cavity with or without a uterus.

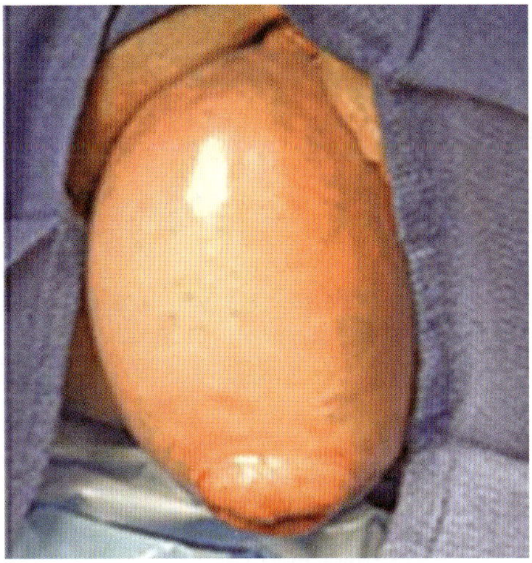

Fig. 1: Le fort partial colpocleisis.

WHY IS IT PERFORMED?

It is indicated only in elderly women who have no future desire for sexual intercourse and having other concomitant medical disorders.

PREOPERATIVE PATIENT EVALUATIONS

Normal Pap smear and normal endometrium either by endometrial biopsy or ultrasonography (USG) is recommended before surgery.

CONSENT

Patient must be fully aware that future vaginal intercourse will not be possible. Risk of procedure about urinary incontinence, urinary retention and sometimes recurrent prolapsed.

SURGICAL STEPS

Anesthesia

Regional or under local anesthesia.

Vaginal Marking

The rectangular areas of vaginal mucosa on anterior and posterior vaginal walls are outline with surgical marker (Figs. 2A and B). Vaginal infiltration inject the vaginal mucosa 50–100 cc normal saline 1:10,000 dilution with adrenalin to

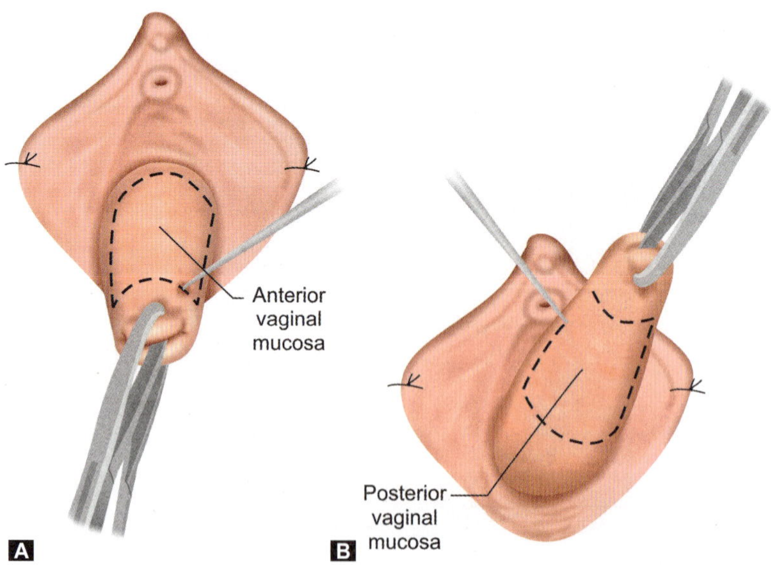

Figs. 2A and B: (A) Anterior vaginal mucosa; (B) Posterior vaginal mucosa.

prevent blood loss and operating field should be clean. The size of rectangular sections or flaps to be removed is determined by the length of vaginal wall. The distal transverse incision should be placed 2 cm above the external os. The proximal transverse incision is made 2–3 cm below the urethral meatus. The width of incision will be determined by the size of the uterus, cervix and vaginal walls.

Vaginal Incisions

Incise the previously marked areas with combination of sharp and blunt dissections. Remove the vaginal epithelium from both anterior & posterior vaginal walls (Figs. 3A and B).

Note: Leave the maximum amount possible for vaginal fibromuscularis on the underlying bladder and rectum. Hemostasis is must. When you remove posterior vaginal flap, avoid entering the peritoneum. If you do open peritoneum, close the defect with delayed absorbable suture.

Stitch the cut edges of anterior and posterior vaginal walls with a row of interrupted stitches with 2-0 delayed absorbable sutures from anterior to posterior distal transverse edges of vagina. These will close the fibromuscular layer over the cervix (Fig. 4).

To replace the uterus into the pelvic cavity, place progressively more caudle rows of interrupted sutures that approximates the anterior and posterior fibro and muscular layer along the width of incision (Fig. 5). Successive transverse tiers of sutures are placed until the proximal transverse vaginal incision is

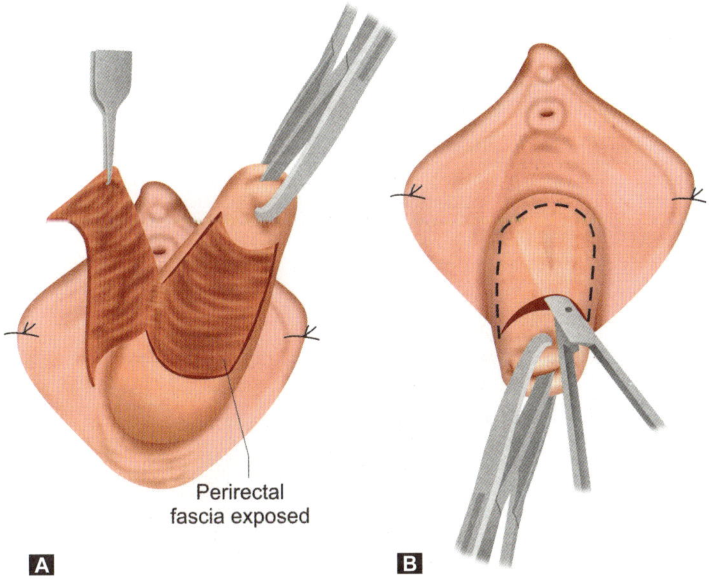

Figs. 3A and B: (A) Anterior vaginal wall; (B) Posterior vaginal wall.

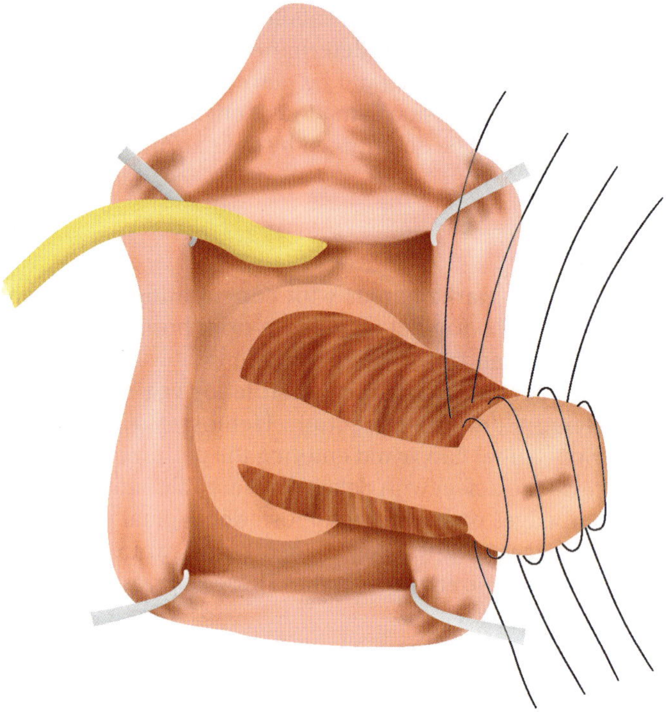

Fig. 4: Stitching the edges with absorbable sutures.

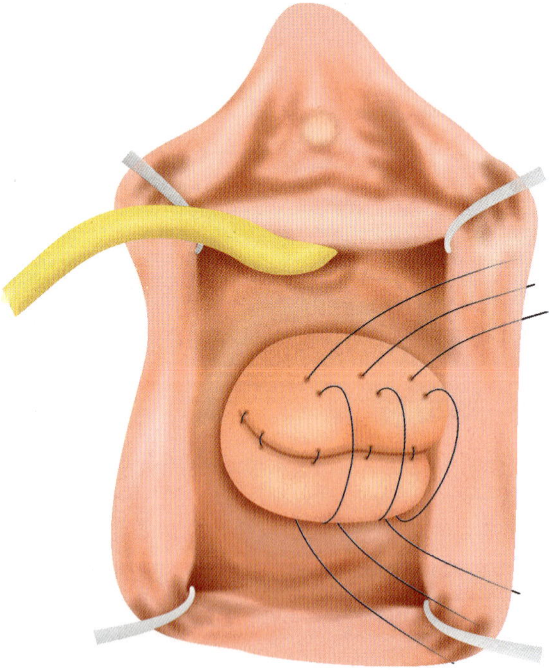

Fig. 5: Placing the transverse tiers of sutures.

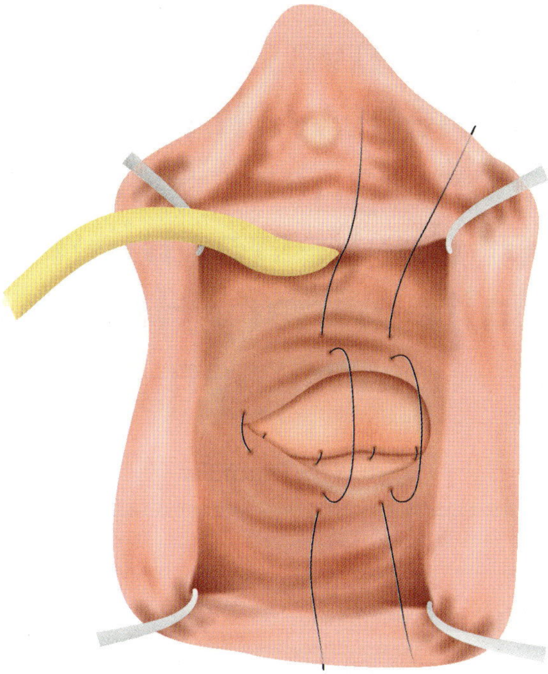

Fig. 6: Closing of vaginal mucosa.

reached. At this point at bladder neck, Kelly placation should be performed to avoid stress urinary incontinence.

The closure of vaginal mucosa

The vaginal mucosa proximal anterior and posterior transverse vaginal edges is closed with two zero delayed absorbable sutures preferably intermittent (Fig. 6).

Postoperative Care

- Perform levator placation and perineorrhaphy as a routine
- Recovery quick and without complications
- Constipation should be avoided
- No heavy lifting at least for 6 weeks.

Chapter 10

Noninvasive Laser Treatment with Functional Electromagnetic Stimulation for the Restoration of Genitourinary Health in Women

Vidya Pancholia

INTRODUCTION

Stress urinary incontinence (SUI) is a major problem in younger women. The main cause is the weakened pelvic floor muscles and connective tissues of the vaginal canal and tissues surrounding the urethra.

This can occur naturally from pregnancy, childbirth, excessive straining, chronic cough, neurologic disorders or just as part of the ageing process or also after gynecological and urological operations.

If these adverse effects are pronounced and prolonged, the position of the bladder can change and even involuntary passage of feces and winds can occur.

Older women more often suffer for an urge urinary incontinence, where urine leaks immediately after an urgent need to urinate.

A large number of women, especially older patients, are faced with a combination of stress and urge incontinence, the so-called mixed urinary incontinence.

About 76% of people consider urinary incontinence as a normal disorder related to aging. However, people with urine leakage problems often feel ashamed and begin to avoid social life. Those people rarely talk about their urine leakage problems, they hide it from their close ones and often also from their doctors. This is why only a few people seek professional help on time.

A nonsurgical treatment, which can be used to prevent and also treat the problem, came in the form of the intensive exercises for the pelvic floor muscles (Kegel exercises), which is only effective with high degree of perseverance which unfortunately usually our women do not seem to have.

Several other therapeutic options are available to alleviate genitourinary syndrome of menopause (GSM) symptoms, including hormonal and nonhormonal products. Moisturizers and lubricants tend to provide only temporary relief, whereas local vaginal estrogen administration offers long-term relief and so is the treatment of choice. However, some women may not wish to take hormone replacement therapy (HRT) long-term or have contraindications to estrogen therapy. Recently ospemifene has been introduced as an oral medication for the treatment of dyspareunia. It provides an alternative to oral and local estrogen therapies. New management strategies for GSM mean that women can choose from a wide range of options, with due consideration to the benefits and risks associated with each.

Another very promising option is laser therapy, which can be used to stimulate tissue repair and to restore normal vaginal function. The word "LASER" is an acronym for "light amplification by stimulated emission of radiation". Lasers generate a beam of photons released from the laser medium; the medium determines the specific wavelength of the light emitted and also typically gives the type of laser its name. Biological tissues such as blood and substances such as melanin and water absorb and react to laser of different wavelengths. Laser treatments use this property of these tissue and substances to safely and effectively offer solutions in many areas, such as dermatology, dentistry, ophthalmology and cosmetic medicine. More recently, several innovative applications on the use of laser in gynecology have also appeared.

Both microablative fractional CO_2 laser and the nonablative vaginal Er:YAG SMOOTH® laser (VEL) used in gynecology induce morphological changes in the vaginal tissues, and data from nonrandomized clinical trials suggest that laser therapy can alleviate vaginal dryness and dyspareunia. VEL has been reported to improve SUI as well as vaginal prolapse by acting upon the tissues in the urogenital area. The erbium-doped yttrium aluminium garnet (Er:YAG) laser uses precisely controlled, sequentially packaged bursts of long pulses, termed SMOOTH® mode (Figs. 1 and 2).

Dr Fistonic and his team demonstrated that the exposure of tissues to an appropriate controlled temperature increase in the range of 60–70°C using VEL in SMOOTH® mode result in a breaking of the intermolecular cross-links that stabilize collagen's triple-helix structure leading to rapid contraction of the

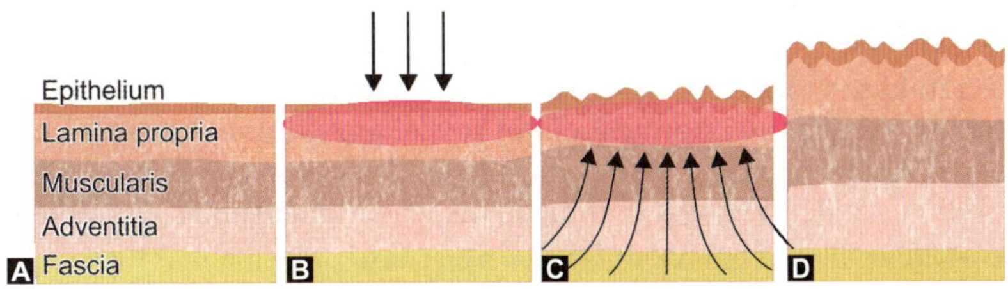

Figs. 1A to D: Mechanism of action of nonablative SMOOTH®-mode erbium laser on the vaginal mucosa: (A) the structure of vaginal mucosa consisting of the epithelium, lamina propria, muscularis, adventitia and fascia; (B) irradiation by special SMOOTH®-mode pulsing sequence of erbium:YAG laser produces collagen hyperthermia in the epithelium and lamina propria; (C) temperature increase to around 65°C on the mucosa surface causes immediate shrinkage of the upper layers of the vaginal wall as well as mechanical pull of the lower lying structures; and (D) 6 months after the treatment there is a significant thickening of the vaginal wall due to new collagen synthesis.

Gomori trichrome stain

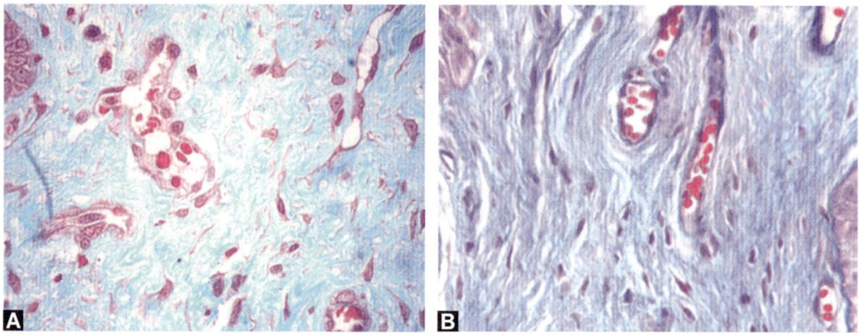

Figs. 2A and B: Pretreatment and post-Er:YAG SMOOTH® Laser treatment—effect on vaginal mucosa. (A) Vaginal mucose sample before IntimaLase® treatment; and (B) Vaginal mucose sample 6 months after IntimaLase® treatment showing increased collagen density.

Courtesy: J Gaviria, MD

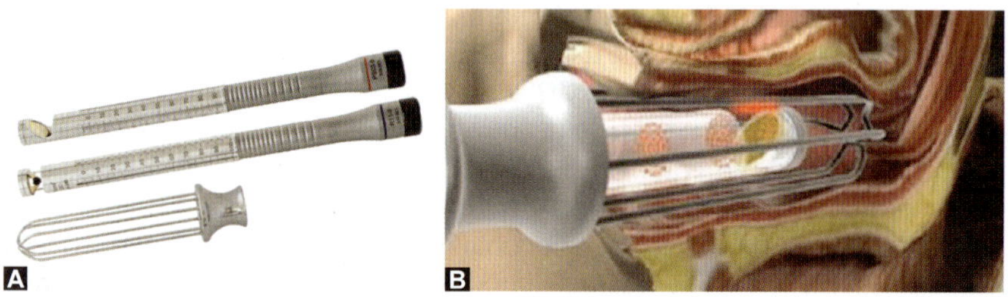

Figs. 3A and B: G-Set accessories needed for application of the erbium:YAG laser beam to the vaginal mucosa, consisting of a laser speculum plus angular and circular adapter.

collagen fibers that in turn results in shrinkage and greater tissue rigidity and also initiating neocollagenesis in vivo. That is, the VEL treatment increased the tissue temperature up to the optimal range (approximately 65°C), but did not exceed the threshold for ablation or irreversible tissue damage. In this way, VEL can increase the density of the connective tissue, stimulating collagen remodeling and neoangiogenesis, leading to a suburethral reinforcement to correct mild to moderate SUI. Furthermore tightening of the vaginal canal and consequently the improvement of sexual gratification have also been observed. Specific vaginal probes have been designed to enable a uniform and well-controlled VEL distribution on the whole length and circumference of the vaginal canal (Figs. 3A and B).

The use of erbium SMOOTH® technology for vaginal tightening nicknamed IntimaLase and stress urinary incontinence, called IncontiLase has spread around the world and many additional studies have been initiated to further assess this technology and treatment approach.

Measurements of an average shrinkage of the vaginal canal after a single IntimaLase treatment, as measured by Dr Rivera, showed 17% shrinkages, while Bezmenko measured an average 56% thickening of the vaginal wall 6 months after two IncontiLase treatments on 77 patients. Using MRI measurements of the shrinkage of the vaginal canal-cross section, Bezmenko and colleagues also demonstrated significant shrinkage of the vaginal canal treated with erbium SMOOTH® technology. The first results from Rivera showed that better results were achieved if a second session of erbium SMOOTH® treatment was additionally performed and his findings were also confirmed by the results of Garcia. Various evaluation tools were used to measure the efficacy of erbium therapy for SUI. Several investigators used the International Consultation on Incontinence Questionnaire-Urinary Incontinence (ICIQ-UI) questionnaires and all found significant reductions in the ICIQ-UI score. Fistonic and colleagues reported a reduction of more than 6 points at 6 months after a single treatment, Gambacciani and Levancini reported more than 6 points of improvement after 3 months and three sessions of erbium therapy. Sencar and Bizjak-Ogrinc reported 77% of SUI patients cured (dry) after 12 months.

The IntimaLase and IncontiLase protocols are based on heating the vaginal wall mucosa up to approximately 65°C and include two treatment sessions with a 4–6-week interval. The time needed to execute the IntimaLase protocol is approximately 8–10 minutes, and for IncontiLase around 15 minutes (as measured by Guimarães). The protocol for treatment of pelvic organ prolapses (ProlapLase) is based on the same principle of collagen hyperthermia as are the protocols for vaginal tightening and incontinence, although with a difference in the treatment intensity (increased) and the location of the major area treated (the prolapsed part of the vaginal wall). The ProlapLase protocol requires 3–5 sessions at 4–6-week intervals. The number of sessions is dependent on the severity (grade) of the prolapse. The vaginal atrophy protocol (RenovaLase) is based on a slightly different concept of milder hyperthermia, whereby the mucosa is warmed up to some 45°C, thus causing the stimulation of cell proliferation via heat shock protein activation, an increase of collagen production as well as anti-inflammatory action. The RenovaLase protocol consists of three sessions at intervals of 3 weeks.

Radiofrequency (RF) is another treatment option designed on the principle of bulk heating of tissue to reach the required temperature in collagen for shrinkage and neocollagenesis. However, RF heats the epithelium to a higher temperature making treatment highly unpleasant. Furthermore use of RF needles necessitates use of anesthetic.

We now also have the possibility for a faster regeneration of muscles and other tissues of the pelvic floor with functional magnetic stimulation (functional magnetic therapy). This therapy replaces and upgrades until now frequently used electrostimulation. In 3–4 weeks with use of magnetic stimulation we can achieve stronger pelvic floor muscles without unpleasant electrode insertion (Fig. 4).

Magnetic therapy has proven to be effective for treatment of all types of urinary incontinence. Because people differ from each other, it is important that the treatment is individualized. For optimum performance throughout the treatment, the program is adopted to the progress. In June 1998, the US Food

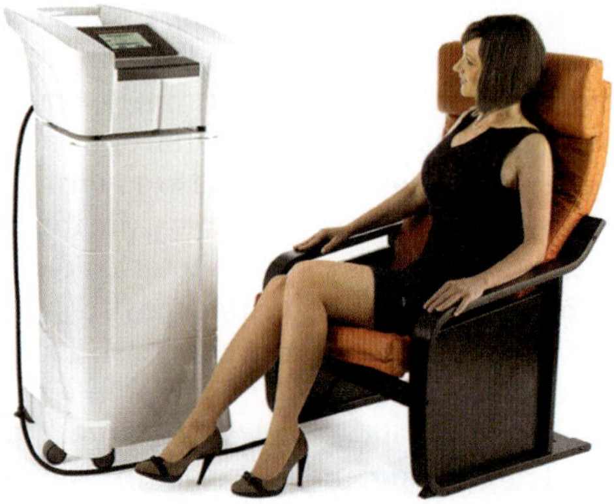

Fig. 4: Treatment of incontinence using a professional device and other issues of the pelvic floor.

and Drug Administration (FDA) recognized functional magnetic stimulation as a conservative method of treatment of urinary incontinence.

The magnetic field generated by the current flow in the coil is proportional to the current passing through it, and the electric field in the tissue is proportional to the rate of change of that magnetic field with respect to time. At the frequencies used in magnetic stimulation the magnetic field is not affect by the electrical properties of the body, and passes through both bone and soft tissue (and even clothing and air) without being affected by them. The magnetic field pulse induces an electric field (a voltage difference between two points) in the tissue which causes an ionic current to flow. If the amplitude, spatial characteristics and duration of this induced current are such that they cause depolarization of a nerve membrane, then stimulation, and the generation of an action potential, will occur (Fig. 5).

Magnetical stimulation of peripheral muscles is achieved via a magnetic stimulation of motor nerves, and not by a direct depolarization of the muscle membrane (Machetanz et al. 1994).

Results of functional magnetic stimulation treatment collected in three centers in 78 female patients treated for urge urinary incontinence (UUI—11 women), mixed urinary incontinence (MUI—23 women), stress urinary incontinence (SUI —30 women) and incontinence after childbirth (14 women). It was noted that almost 90% of women with UUI, MUI and SUI reported a significant improvement with almost 75% of SUI cases and 60% of UUI and MUI cases becoming fully dry. In the post childbirth incontinence 100% of women were fully dry post-treatment.

During the therapy, patients are sitting dressed in a comfortable chair and a treatment is carried out twice or three times a week for 20 minutes. In the absence of direct contact with the skin, the treatment is not painful or uncomfortable and has no known side effects.

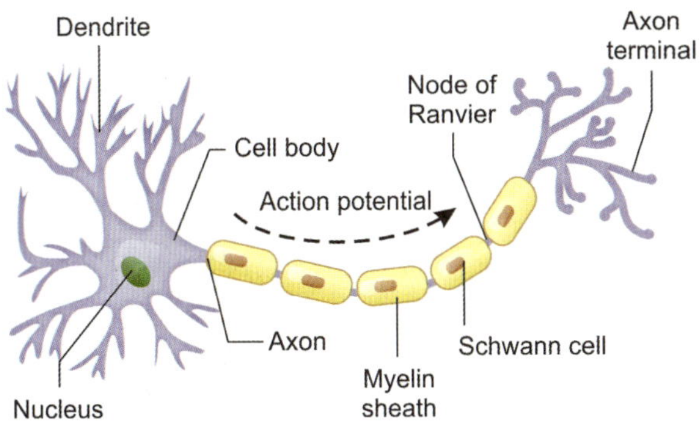

Fig. 5: Structure of neuron.

CONCLUSION

We believe that the noninvasive erbium:YAG SMOOTH® laser can be combined with the functional magnetic stimulation for an efficacious and safe new method for the treatment of vaginal laxity, stress urinary incontinence, pelvic organ prolapses, and vaginal atrophy. The VEL and FMS combine beautifully to treat tissue and muscle disorders and this type of combined therapy will soon become the treatment of choice for these indications.

BIBLIOGRAPHY

1. Gambacciani M, Palacios P. Laser therapy for the restoration of vaginal function. Maturitas. 2017;99:10-5.
2. Portman DJ, Gass ML, Vulvovaginal atrophy Terminology Consensus Conference Panel. Genitourinary syndrome of menopause: new terminology for vulvovaginal atrophy from the International Society for the Study of Women's Sexual Health and the North American Menopause Society. Climateric. 2014;17(5):557-63.
3. Štrumbelj T, Podnar P, Mežek ZK, et al. Treatment of uncontrolled urine leakage problems. Derma Hair Journal. 2014;49.